In the Mind Fields

In the Mind Fields

Exploring the New Science of Neuropsychoanalysis

Casey Schwartz

PANTHEON BOOKS, NEW YORK

All rights reserved. Published in the United States by Pantheon Books,
a division of Penguin Random House LLC, New York, and in Canada by Random House
of Canada, a division of Penguin Random House Ltd., Toronto.

Pantheon Books and colophon are registered trademarks of
Penguin Random House LLC.

This is a work of nonfiction, but the names of certain individuals as well as identifying
descriptive details concerning them have been changed to protect their privacy.

Library of Congress Cataloging-in-Publication Data
Schwartz, Casey.
In the mind fields: exploring the new science of neuropsychoanalysis / Casey Schwartz.
pages cm
ISBN 978-0-307-91152-0 (hardcover : alk. paper). ISBN 978-0-307-91153-7 (eBook).
1. Neuropsychiatry. 2. Psychoanalysis. 3. Neuropsychology. 4. Cognitive neuroscience.
I. Title.
RC341.S336 2015 616.89'17—DC23 2014046677

www.pantheonbooks.com

Jacket design by Janet Hansen
Book design by Maggie Hinders

Printed in the United States of America
First Edition

2 4 6 8 9 7 5 3 1

For my parents, for Adam & for Ellen,
with love

INTRODUCTION

I'd never been a science person. I didn't relate at all. So it was with a sense of surprise, a year out of college, that I discovered I loved studying the brain. I was enrolled at UCLA summer school, trying to cobble together the necessary academic credits to apply for graduate school in psychology, the field I thought I wanted to enter. On the list of requirements was a class called Behavioral Neuroscience. I was surprised to see it included there. A decade earlier, it might not have been. But there had been a groundswell in neuroscience in recent years, beginning in the early 1990s, and the field was now an undeniable force in the struggle to clarify and define human mental life. Understanding the brain had become *de rigueur* for those who wanted to understand the mind. It was another side to the story.

"Biology is truly a land of unlimited possibilities. We may expect it to give us the most surprising information, and we cannot guess what answers it will return in a few dozen years to the questions we have put to it. They may be of a kind that will blow away the whole of our artificial structure of hypotheses." So reflected Sigmund Freud in 1920, more than three decades after the great turning point of his working life: from hard science to the "purely psychological." Back then, in the mid-1880s, he had been toiling away in labs, peering down microscopes, for going on twenty years. But he would soon arrive at the conclusion that the questions he wanted to answer about the human mind couldn't be answered by what was then understood—or understandable—about the human brain. The knowledge wasn't there and neither were the tools. So he would work with what was available: mental life, in all of its manifestations. He continued to emphasize, however, that eventually, long after his own lifetime, the moment would come when brain science would be ready to fill out the psychoanalytic principles of the mind he was busy laying down.

There are some who believe that moment is here. Yet it's doubtful that even Freud could have anticipated just how far apart the two disciplines have grown. Psychoanalysis and neuroscience, with their starkly different goals, methods, and cultures, can appear to be two different species, mutually alienated, as if preoccupied with two altogether different pursuits. In our current moment, the terrain is uneven. Psychoanalysis is a field under siege; neuroscience is the golden child, commanding newspaper headlines, substantial government grants, and an ever-increasing portion of the public imagination. The brain has become our modern metaphor: it is the repository of truth, it is where we look to find out what's *really* going on. Already, neuroscientific research has penetrated the field of economics, the courts, and beyond. It animates ongoing debates about how our evolving understanding of the brain should affect models of decision making, how it should be taken into account in the carrying out of legal justice. It is decidedly less common to hear psychoanalytic concepts invoked in these same circles.

Despite the real schism between these two fields, there are a growing number of people—analysts, scientists, and others—who are attempting to build a bridge between them, however unlikely the idea, however unimaginable the design. In no sense could this movement be described as mainstream. The word *fringe* is batted about. Nevertheless, the very struggle to bring some of the old ideas about the mind into the new landscape of the brain is one I believe to be both worthwhile and revealing.

It is a struggle I stumbled upon accidentally, when I entered graduate school with the intention of becoming a psychologist. But it wasn't until afterwards, when I'd set aside that goal and become instead the person with the tape recorder observing from the sidelines, that I could finally see the extent of the efforts, the setbacks, the stakes.

It all began so innocently. In the din of the hallway that led to our high school cafeteria my friend Katia, aspiring actress, aged sixteen, turned to me to remark: "That's *so* Freudian."

I chuckled. Paused. Then asked the question I'd been wondering about on some level for years, listening in on all the New York conversations where the subject, in one way or another, came up. "By the way, what exactly does that mean?"

"Oh, you know, it's when you repress things into your unconscious," she said.

I would gain no further clarity until I was a sophomore in college, enrolled in a course called Literature and Psychoanalysis. Finally, I was going to understand the mysterious terms I'd heard forever, particles in the cultural ether: *the unconscious, the conscious, the ego, the id.* I believe we started with *Civilization and Its Discontents.* It was a crowd-pleaser. I didn't know that yet. I was happy to be pleased, to be dazzled, by Freud's radical imagining of the mind.

Against the dulled or vulgar or simplified surface of things, he offered the tantalizing promise of subtext, a deeper truth, a further realm. He dared to challenge the constructions people offered up about themselves; he had the nerve, and the wit, to trace backwards through the years from, let's say, the pinched and upstanding adult to the child unduly fascinated by his own "excreta," as Freud puts it. There was a humor in all this, a taste for the absurd, and a blessed lack of squeamishness. Everyone—fetishists, onanists, and inverts alike—found a home in Freud's interested gaze. Of course, there were painful moments of Freud on women. His dismissiveness at these times was hard to bear, as much for its failure of imagination as anything else. But I could get past it. His ideas about the human mind were like majestic carpets rolled out to cover vast, empty spaces.

One afternoon, four years later, plunged into Behavioral Neuroscience at UCLA, I noticed that our teaching assistant, a doctoral student named Eric, seemed deflated. "Everyone please come stand around this table," he said. He was wearing latex gloves. We gathered around and looked down into a bucket with chemical-smelling liquid swishing inside, from which Eric was suddenly pulling out a brain, holding it up on one flat palm.

"Is that a *human* brain?" I said. I was confused by my classmates' collective reaction. They were unmoved. They were bored.

"Yes!" Eric said, perking up, "and all day everyone's been acting like they don't understand how amazing this is."

Eric balanced the brain as delicately as if it were a newborn. I stared at it, at its shocking, intestine-like wrinkles, which, in the chemical bath, had turned the color of dirty snow. Its sheer exoticism bordered on the obscene. I did not identify with this object.

Later I would learn that the shock of unfamiliarity I was feeling is actually a feature of the brain. The brain is inclined to make itself unknown, producing for each of us a version of reality that feels objective, but is in fact utterly subjective, varying among us for myriad reasons—mood, intelligence, experience, genetics. Because of the brain's built-in tendency to remain behind the scenes, we're not aware that so many elements of our daily lives—even, perhaps, every single one—are subject to interpretation.

Yet here, in Psych. 115, I was learning that neuroscience disdains, above all, subjective interpretations. It traffics in hard truth, empirical data, conclusions demonstrable in a laboratory. There is a machismo to the pursuit, both in its no-nonsense ethos and in its pioneering quality, eager researchers charging out into uncharted land.

"Let's say it's Saturday night and we want to take a little amphetamine," our professor, Brian Armstrong, began. This was apparently a standard opening line in a neuroscience class. And in any neuroscience class, even the most innocent, which ours surely was not—the subject of drugs is going to come up often and in great detail. In fact, it is from looking at how different drugs—cannabis, opiates, alcohol, speed, you name it, they've studied it—affect the brain that scientists have discerned its naturally occurring neurotransmitters, the pathways they operate on, and the effects they have.

"Why would you want to get off Prozac? It's delicious," said Pro-

fessor Armstrong in class one day. During another lecture, in order
to illustrate the concept that each hemisphere of the brain picks
up signals from the opposite half of the body, Professor Armstrong
remarked that if, hypothetically, he were to "take a buzz saw to your
left inner thighs," it would be the right half of our brains that would
hear about it.

It was high drama. It was all very vivid. It was not a bad way to
begin.

One year later, I arrived in London, enrolled in a brand-new master's program, a two-year course divided between the Anna Freud
Centre in London and Yale the following year. The idea was to
combine psychoanalysis and neuroscience: one year immersed in
classic masterworks of psychoanalytic theory, followed by a second
year devoted to studying the brain and to working in the labs of
Yale's cutting-edge neuroscientists. The program's hybrid shape
seemed like a chance to survey the fields devoted to the mind and
to the brain, to begin to understand what was happening on both
ends of the spectrum. My classmates and I—there were only nine
of us—would be the first group to go through. We were the trial
balloon.

It was an unlikely undertaking. These two disciplines, psychoanalysis and neuroscience, were mostly indifferent to each other,
and even, as I would learn, at times opposed. Psychology, as a field,
has gone through countless overhauls and identity crises since Freud
began asking his patients to lie down on the couch. As the study of
the mind, psychology is by definition ephemeral, a search for insight
and improvement difficult to capture with charts and graphs. This
was an understanding that Freud and the psychoanalysts who fol-

lowed him embraced. They studied inner reality, psychic conflicts, dynamic forces, repressed material, defense mechanisms. They made careful and detailed records of their patients' free associations, tracking progress and regressions. They followed a systematic approach, but there is a limitation to how empirical psychoanalysis can be. Many—maybe most—are unwilling to call it a science.

It's not easy to wedge the two fields into coherent study. Psychoanalysis wielded an enormous authority throughout the twentieth century, and continues to influence our most basic assumptions about human nature. The power of the unconscious mind, the profound importance of early childhood experience in shaping the course of our lives—these are but two of the discoveries originally advanced by psychoanalysts and now considered indispensable to our understanding, psychological, cultural, and otherwise, of both the mind and the brain. Yet, by the 1950s, the enthusiasm for the new cognitive sciences prompted a feeling, a concern, among many American psychoanalysts especially, that their own field would never be fully legitimate without something concrete to measure, without recourse to the scientific method, in all of its *if this then that* clarity and rigor. When I arrived in London in 2006, a form of this anxiety continued to bubble up around me.

Recently, I decided to investigate the roots of the long, occasionally ambiguous quest that began for me in London and continued on to New Haven, New York, Montreal, Washington, D.C., Cape Town, and Paris, through psychoanalytic offices and neuroscientific labs, to conference halls and hospital bedsides. After hours spent digging through my mother's basement, I finally came up with them: my old college notebooks. I opened the white spiral I had kept for Literature and Psychoanalysis class. There, on the first page, in notes taken down during lecture, the Freudian story began:

with the iconic case of Anna O., the young Viennese woman who brought her hysterical symptoms for treatment in the early 1880s and, as she began to improve, referred to the treatment process as her "talking cure." It was with a sense of shock that I registered the date at the top of the page: September 13, 2001.

More than ten years later, I can't say whether those old, rich, foundational ideas about the mind seemed especially vital, even crucial, at a moment in time when so many things had suddenly stopped making sense. I only know that a semi-straight line exists between that day in September and another September day, five years later, when I arrived in London to join the Freudians in the passionate and elevated atmosphere I imagined they inhabited.

So began my journey through the world of the mind, the brain, and the elusive territory that might be described as somewhere in between. This book is a record of that trip.

PART ONE

1

---

20 Maresfield Gardens
London, N.W. 3
Nov. 28th, 1938

Dear H.D.,
  I got today some flowers. By chance or intention they are my
favourite flowers, those I most admire. Some words 'to greet the
return of the God' (other people read: Goods). No name. I suspect
you to be responsible for the gift. If I have guessed right don't
answer but accept my hearty thanks for so charming a gesture.
In any case,

Affectionately yours,
Sigm. Freud

FALL 2006

In North London, just around the corner from Maresfield Gardens, there is a bronze statue of Freud at the base of the hill that starts at Swiss Cottage and slopes up to Hampstead. Freud is seated, but barely: he is leaning forward, in a vitalized, even agitated state, as if about to leap to his feet and pounce on you with his discerning insight. When I arrived in London to begin graduate school, I understood this statue to be a notification of sorts: I had passed into Freud World. I was on his turf now.

My classes were held at the Anna Freud Centre, a narrow red-and-white brick building, formerly a private residence, like most of the houses on this leafy, self-enclosed street. Anna and her father, an ailing Sigmund Freud, were installed just across the street when they arrived in London in 1938, fleeing Nazi-occupied Vienna. Freud died the next year. But Anna stayed on in the house on Maresfield Gardens. She opened the center during World War II, as a clinic for children. She would remain the de facto international leader of psychoanalysis until her own death in 1982.

She may or may not have been her father's favorite daughter, but she was the one he brought into the family business. He analyzed her himself, in sporadic bursts between 1918 and 1925. Anna, like her father, was veiled and resolute, but lacked his expansive, metaphorical touch. In written accounts, she is distinctly no-nonsense. Most believe that Anna Freud's writing never equaled her father's depth and passion. "This is because—I'm sorry to say it—she was a woman; she was not a genius. When a genius writes, there is always so much more, and it is open to the whole world," Kurt Eissler, the former director of the Sigmund Freud Archives, once told the journalist Janet Malcolm. Yet Anna Freud would enter history as one of the pioneers of the new, growing field of child psychology.

In psychoanalytic institutes around the world, Freud is read in a fairly specific order. At the Anna Freud Centre, the order in which we proceeded through Freud's work was all the more prescribed. The crucial thing, we learned, was to trace his thought process, from its beginnings in the last decade of the nineteenth century to its final form, along all the diversions and revisions and lost causes in between.

Throughout our first term in London, Dr. Nick Midgley, understated and aristocratic, a child analyst and scholar on Freud, guided us through the fundamental analytic texts. Freud, who struggled to successfully hypnotize his patients, abandoned the method quickly, but preserved the idea of creating a hypnotic air, a quiet, hushed, liberated place where patients could reach new limits within their own minds. We were launched into Vienna, 1895, where women were seized with hysterias, alleging sexual abuses.

I wondered about all the hysterical patients Freud described and the florid symptoms they suffered—fleeting paralyses, the sudden inability to speak, the nagging presence of untraceable odors. There was a mystery here, which was rarely addressed. The question puzzled me in its obviousness: Where were these hysterics now? How could any condition evidently so widespread in fin de siècle Europe exist only in that time and place? Had the root cause somehow disappeared over the years, or was it that the condition had transformed into modern versions, maybe something like anorexia or borderline personality disorder? Somehow, I didn't manage to get an answer.

To become a practicing psychoanalyst, one must travel down a long, mysterious road. We were on the outskirts, peering in, contending with the strange new vocabulary with which analysts have fitted out the human psyche. "We encourage you to purchase the psychoanalytic dictionary," we were told soon after we began our classes. "It's available at Karnac Books, on the Finchley Road." To get to the Finchley Road, one descended as if from a dreamscape,

dropping down the sharply slanted hill that connected the time-
less tranquility of Maresfield Gardens to the busy commerce of the
high street below. I entered Karnac to discover the shrine to all texts
psychoanalytic, the store shrouded in a respectful hush. I thumbed
through the erudite selection. In the months to come, when in Karnac, I would creep around the edges. I wouldn't make a sound. On
this inaugural foray, I located the dictionary and shuffled away with
my purchase.

As suggested by the very fact of a dictionary, psychoanalytic
language is often opaque and maddeningly ambiguous. There is a
term for everything that happens in the realm of the conscious, the
preconscious, and the unconscious. There are reaction formations,
repressions, and resistances. *Phantasy* is not to be confused with *fantasy*. Ditto *imago:* no mere image. The issue of the psychoanalytic
vocabulary is complicated by the fact that a single term has different
meanings, depending on which camp you belong to. *Countertransference* means one thing to a Freudian, and another to a Kleinian.
The difference, both sides will tell you, is not negligible. Freud had
a phrase that perfectly captures the situation: the narcissism of small
differences. He first presented the idea in my old favorite, *Civilization and Its Discontents:*

> I once discussed the phenomenon that it is precisely communities
> with adjoining territories, and related to each other in other ways
> as well, who are engaged in constant feuds and ridiculing each
> other—like the Spaniards and the Portuguese, for instance, the
> North Germans and South Germans, the English and Scotch,
> and so on. I gave this phenomenon that name of the "narcis-
> sism of minor differences," a name which does not do much to
> explain it.

. . .

A certain suspension of disbelief was required, I soon found, to enter Freud's world. It was a place of neither fact nor fiction. For this reason, it was jolting to see patients arrive at the Anna Freud Centre for their analytic sessions. They were living, breathing humans, commuting to and from North London; not far-away governesses suffering from unheard-of symptoms. When they were early, they would sit in the stiff wooden chairs arranged on each landing, next to small tables stacked with back issues of *The New Yorker.*

Neuroscience, with its strict demand—*prove it*—was hardly mentioned during our first months in London. The very absence of scientific proof in psychoanalysis, the very impossibility of it, has indelibly shaped the field. Without the cool detachment of the scientific method to prune wrong from right, to falsify or not, psychoanalytic theories began to sprawl in divergent directions through the decades following Freud's first sessions. To this day, there are countless schools of thought within psychoanalytic thought, numerous irreconcilable differences.

The chief example of the legacy of disagreement is perhaps embodied in the figure of Melanie Klein. In my imagining, Klein cut a sinister figure in the history of psychoanalysis. Black associations swirled around her: obsessions with hatred, rage, and envy. Her unhappy childhood in Vienna, where she experienced herself as the least wanted of all her siblings. Later, trapped in an unsatisfying life with small children of her own, Klein found her way to *The Interpretation of Dreams,* just published, and through it to the new science of psychoanalysis.

As Nick Midgley struggled to explain over the course of the first semester, the essence of the theoretical divide that would open up

between the Freudians and the Kleinians came down to the Oedipus complex. Freud believed that the Oedipal crisis—the desire
for the mother, the terror of the father's revenge—was the seminal
moment in childhood development. Starting at age three or four,
Freud writes, the child must devise a solution to the threat he per-
ceives from his vengeful father, on whom he depends for survival.
The child opts to identify with his father, a decision that inaugurates
the child's conscience, the internalizing of his father's own store of
values and sense of what ought to be. But Klein, in her sessions
with very young children, believed that even in earliest infancy, well
before the challenge of the Oedipal stage, babies grapple with psychic conflict, intense feelings of aggression, frustration, hatred, and
envy; that they have a major developmental task to deal with far
earlier than Freud believed: they have to reconcile everything they
love and everything they hate about their mother, to see that these
all belong to one single object, and advance beyond the view of the
world around them as being split between "good" and "bad." Klein
would later add more distinctions to her ideas about infancy, but it
was her concept of the pre-Oedipal phase that marked the dividing
line between her own followers and the Freudians.

Here's Freud, in a 1927 letter to the analyst Ernest Jones: "The
opinions of Frau Klein about the behavior of the ego ideal with
children seem absolutely impossible to me and are in complete contradiction to all my basic assumptions." More than a decade later,
Anna Freud would still be doing battle with Klein and her followers.
In 1940, as London reeled from German bombs, Anna Freud and
Melanie Klein dug into their respective positions. They repeatedly
debated each other in front of an audience of colleagues at the British Psychoanalytical Society. These debates have come to be known
as the "Controversial Discussions." Ultimately, the two camps went

their separate ways, Klein's ideas laying the foundation for the British object relations school, dominant to this day.

An irony I would never quite parse: despite the acrimony that had rived the British analytic community, the Kleinians made their headquarters not even two blocks away from the Anna Freudians', at the Tavistock, a big boxy structure of poured concrete, a postwar lummox amid the elegant houses on Fitzjohn's Avenue. Walking by on my way to class, I would stare through the curtainless windows into rooms of Kleinians-in-training, sitting in circular formations. I had the beguiling sense of spying on the enemy.

From time to time, throughout the year in London, a Kleinian arrived from the Tavistock to deliver a guest lecture at the Anna Freud Centre. It was always something of an occasion. On one such afternoon, a Kleinian analyst arrived to present a recent case. My classmates and I, squeezed into our metal chairs, entered into the contemplative lull we had by then learned to cultivate, a layman's version of the "evenly hovering attention" that analysts are trained to employ. Our speaker began. She had, in the last two years, been seeing a young woman who, we were told, arrived for every session, regardless of the season, regardless of the weather, dressed in pants. Never skirts, never dresses, only pants. The analyst paused to let us absorb this apparently meaningful detail.

"Finally," she said, "I made my interpretation. It had become clear that she was repulsed by her own genitals."

There was a silence in the room.

I raised my hand. "Could there really be no other explanation?"

The speaker looked at me with an expression of surprise at the very question.

"No," she said. "It was her genital repulsion."

And that was that. Somehow, perhaps unfairly, this moment

lodged in my mind as quintessentially Kleinian: a taking of liberties with one's intuitions, a reckless foray into the realm of pure speculation, laced with real aggression. It had begun with Klein's daring to interpret the psychological struggles unfolding inside the tiny skulls of preverbal infants. Now here we were in 2006, drawing bizarre and potentially damaging conclusions. I was extremely uncomfortable. Of course, I too wore pants, only pants.

———

The last thing we were assigned to read before Christmas was Freud's evocative watershed paper "Mourning and Melancholia." In this dense work, Freud puzzles over the question of depression, though he doesn't call it that, and what makes melancholia different from mourning. I fell into the text, taking in Freud's formulations. Both mourning and melancholia, Freud says, are, to begin with, states of withdrawal from the world, and both are prompted by some real, external loss.

The paper is short but it brims with ideas that changed the course of psychoanalytic theory in the years to follow. It is considered the work that led to the concept of the superego, the third and final layer of Freud's so-called metapsychology. But in truth, it was not this breakthrough in the mapping of the mental structure that most grasped my interest. I was thinking of my father.

As I was reading Freud's essay, my father, a novelist and radio personality, was mired in depression, debilitated almost beyond recognition, for what had then been nearly three years. I had last seen him on my twenty-fourth birthday, two weeks before I left for London, for graduate school. My mother and father had both flown from New York to California, where I lived at the time, to celebrate this birthday with me. It was a disaster. I saw that my father, off the plane, was unreachable, a person in another dimension.

That night, we went to a boxing match in downtown Los Angeles. David, the boyfriend I lived with, was an obsessive boxing fan and it seemed the natural way to spend the evening. David and my brother Adam and my chic mother in her black cashmere uniform and my walking corpse of a father and I all sat in a row and watched two heavyweight champions, Sam "The Nigerian Nightmare" Peter and James "Lights Out" Toney, throw their punches and dance the ring and fall into those intermittent embraces that boxers use for rest, as well as for moments of closeness, it always seemed to me.

No one was really able to watch the fight. That's how it is when you're sitting next to a zombie. It is not the case that the zombie recedes into invisibility, that his presence is forgotten. Anyone who has been around a person trapped in deep depression knows all about this. Your life, too, must shrink down to those tiny, miserable parameters.

My father murmured that he was going to get a hot dog and lurched to his feet. The rest of us looked at one another nervously. "Are you okay?" my mother asked him. Long divorced, they had always remained close friends. "Of course, of course," he said, aiming for levity. I wasn't sure that he would be able to make it back. The author of five books and a presence on American radio for forty years could not be relied upon to make a trip to the hot dog stand.

Well, he returned, with sauerkraut.

After the fight, we went for Korean barbecue. The restaurant was a favorite, but the atmosphere remained grim. I had the image of my father as an abused child, his presence a mere cobweb at the table. Do I need to explain that my father was not always like this? Do I need to say something here about how he was, for all the years

I'd known him, wild, hilarious, colorful, eccentric, electric? Sometimes very black, too, but always, always a heavyweight. And yet, evidently, this was still my father, this person at the table whose uncomprehending eyes stared vaguely in my direction through the gusts of steam rising from our plates.

There had been clues. For a while now, he'd been doing this falling thing, this thing where suddenly, without warning, he would fall, extravagantly, onto the floor. He did it on the street, he did it in the elevator, he did it in lobbies and in restaurants. He never hurt himself, and it wasn't neurological, doctors told him. Later, I would think of him when I was studying Freud's hysterics, whose limbs were apt to give out at inexplicable moments.

There was another moment, too. I was home in New York for my brother's high school graduation. We were all there, the stepparents and half siblings, and it was a happy occasion, watching Adam, the beloved punk, cross the stage to get his diploma while noticeably chewing gum.

Out on the street afterwards, my father turned to me.

"My God," he said, "I can't figure out where the car is."

"Where'd you park it?"

"That's not it," he said, looking left towards Park Avenue and right towards Lexington. "I can't figure out which is east and which is west."

My father had lived almost his whole life in Manhattan, in most cases mere blocks from where we stood.

And then California. At the end of the gloomy evening, which I had largely spent in tears, we dropped my father off first, then drove my mother to her hotel on La Cienega. I got out of the car to hug her good night. I believed I had ruined the whole night that she'd tried so hard to infuse with festivity. Flying west, bearing presents, ordering cakes, and being, as ever, full of enthusiasm and brightness for the future. But my mother just grabbed me and said, "It's awful, isn't it?"

Through the first months in London, I still spoke to my father occasionally, but the calls were tedious and detached and I couldn't wait to hang up. His availability had always been subject to change. Now it was simply gone.

In "Mourning and Melancholia," Freud describes how the ego is born into the world prepared to attach itself to people around it. *Cathexis* is the word Freud used to denote this attachment. The ego, Freud says, sticks its cathexis onto love objects of its choosing. At first the ones that happen to be there; later, a more select group.

In melancholia, Freud says, what seems to be happening is that this love object, the one with the cathexis stuck onto it, gets lost, goes away, rejects you, disappoints you. You withdraw your cathexis back into the ego, now that there's nothing there anymore for it to stick to. But what happens once the ego turns back in on itself is less straightforward. "In mourning it is the world which has become poor and empty," Freud writes. "In melancholia, it is the ego itself." There is, Freud says, the persistent sense that *something* is missing.

In my father's case, I knew only too well who the lost object was that had sent him into his three-year coma. Her name was Liese, she was thirty-three to his sixty-five, and she'd finally ended things between them. He'd been involved with her for a decade, now, throughout much of his marriage to my stepmother. Why did I even know about this? Well, I did. My father had taken me into his confidence years before. Liese lived in a little studio apartment on West End Avenue, where she kept an embroidered cloth over her television when she wasn't using it. "She thinks someone could see her through the screen," my father told me. "What's wrong with that?" I'd been to the apartment. I'd seen the cloth.

The situation played out in my mind as I read through Freud's essay. I put it down. I picked it up. Read it again. Suddenly, my eyes focused on a short passage, near the beginning. It was one of those plot twists that stop the heart, that run throughout Freud's whole forty years of writing. It is just a single observation:

> One cannot see clearly what it is that has been lost, and it is all the more reasonable to suppose that the patient cannot consciously perceive what he has lost either. This, indeed, might be so even if the patient is aware of the loss which has given rise to his melancholia, but only in the sense that he knows *whom* he has lost but not *what* he has lost in him.

The loss is unknown. I scribbled it in the margin. *The loss is unknown.* Underlined it three times. I had never before considered that maybe my father didn't know exactly what the loss was that had so capsized him. That maybe he was as hopelessly estranged from his own mind at that moment as I was from him. If that were true, then we were estranged together, a little bit closer than I'd thought.

I went back to New York for Christmas break and, almost immediately, broke my foot while riding on the back of a friend's Vespa. It was a Vespa I didn't want to be on in the first place. It was late at night and the pedals were strangely ambiguous. We turned up a side street and before I realized it, we were accelerating into the narrow passage between moving traffic and parked cars. In one instant, my right foot crunched up against a wall of metal, my bones snapping like fresh carrot sticks. We zipped to the hospital. Next to us in the triage area, a drunk woman missing the outer layer of her face was waiting for a doctor. She'd fallen down a flight of stairs at a bar.

"Aging's a bitch," she kept remarking in a raspy voice. As we waited for the X-ray, my mind flashed to images of the coming months: navigating through London on crutches, the crowded Tube, the long stretch of rain-slicked avenue that led to school. I passed the rest of the holiday horizontally, lying in my childhood bedroom, captive to the household routines for the first time since high school. My mood swayed from sullen to stricken. I scooted up and down the stairs on my ass. I had lost my clarity.

After Freud's death, the principles of practicing psychoanalysis became, in the Anglo-American world at least, stricter, more literal-minded, every point carried out to a painstaking degree: the unbudging fifty-minute hour; the extreme impersonality—the "mask-like blankness"—cultivated by the purists of the profession. All had begun as suggestions that became rules that became dogma. And so, too, the enduring portrait of Freud constricted into something much more rigid and aloof than the man himself ever was.

I was confused—disheartened, in fact—by this development. I continued to think of Freud in much different terms; I continued to think of him as the character I had first encountered years before, when I'd read a short, somewhat obscure book called *Tribute to Freud,* by the American poet and writer known as H.D., who had been one of his patients. I came to the book as an undergraduate, but returned to it periodically, each time drawn in anew by its peculiar, dreamlike intensity.

H.D. went off to Vienna in 1933 to begin her work with "the Professor." At that time, she was forty-seven years old. She had earned an international reputation from her work. She had been Ezra Pound's lover. She wasn't any longer. It was Pound who had bequeathed her the initials, spontaneously signing "H. D. Imagiste" at the end of one of her early poems, thereby banishing "Hilda Doolittle."

When it was offered to her, she said yes right away. How could she not accept the chance to be analyzed by Sigmund Freud? Everyone knew he had only a few years left to live. Early in the spring of 1933, H.D. checked into the Hotel Regina, where she would stay for the duration of her analysis. But when she got to 19 Berggasse for her first appointment, she was struck by a terrible sense of self-consciousness: What was the etiquette for one's first appearance in this iconic sanctuary? She gave her coat to the girl who greeted her and waited nervously in the outer chamber of Freud's office. "I know that Prof. Dr. Sigmund Freud will open the door which faces me. Although I know this and have been preparing for some months for this ordeal, I am, nonetheless, taken aback, surprised, shocked even, when the door opens," she writes. "He appears too suddenly."

In a state of numbed uncertainty, H.D. walked through his door. "He is waiting for me to say something. I cannot speak." Instead, she looked around, taking in all his famous objects, his little ancient statues and wrought-iron figurines.

"You are the only person who has ever come into this room and looked at the things in the room before looking at me," Freud said.

The moment had been fumbled. When Freud's little lion dog came running up, H.D. bent down to greet her, glad for the diversion. "Yofi—her name is Yofi—snuggles her nose into my hand and nuzzles her head, in delicate sympathy, against my shoulder," she would write.

Yet soon, right away, they were past all that. In some sense, they already knew each other. Freud had ordered all of H.D.'s books sent to him in advance, so that by the time she turned up for their sessions, he'd read everything she'd published.

Freud, I couldn't help noticing, had taken her seriously as a writer. Indeed, the question of her gender had not seemed to intrude much upon their dynamic at all. Except, perhaps, for a single queer moment. Late one afternoon, towards the end of their session, Freud was suddenly pounding his fist on the headpiece of the horsehair sofa she lay on. "The trouble is—I am an old man," he told her. *"You do not think it worth your while to love me."*

H.D. did not know what the provocation had been. She smoothed out the little rug that had fallen to the floor, trying to hide her discomfort. "My mind was detached enough to wonder if this was some idea of *his* for speeding up the analytic content or redirecting the flow of associated images," she writes. Then: "He must know everything or he didn't know anything."

With Freud, she discussed her childhood in Pennsylvania, her inscrutable astronomer father who slept all day, her mother, her brother who died fighting in the First World War. Years later, she wondered whether to write about the analysis. She feared it would be gratuitous, that there were already so many others who would write their own versions among Freud's lustrous patients, like the man whose sessions preceded hers, whom she'd always admired when she passed him on the stairs, the man widely known, Freud had told her, as "the flying Dutchman." But he crashed his plane in Tanganyika. Finally, H.D. swatted away her self-doubt, deciding: "It is easy to say, 'Everybody will be scribbling memoirs,' but the answer to that is, 'Indeed yes, but neither the Princess George of Greece nor Dr. Hanns Sachs aforetime of Vienna and Berlin, later of Boston, Massachusetts, can scribble exactly *my* impressions of the Professor.'"

Tribute to Freud shows a Freud who is moody, chatty, convivial. He gossips; he writes spry, affectionate notes to his patients, thanking them for gifts, checking in, making jokes; he strolls out into the waiting room to continue a conversation; he is given to suddenly declaring, "Ah—now—we must celebrate *this*," when his patient has said something that strikes him, then carefully choosing and lighting a fresh cigar to mark the occasion. This Freud, I recognized. This was the Freud I knew. So where had he gone, this Freud of my heart, who I'd first known and loved as a student of literature in my undergraduate days? I'd followed him to London and he'd disappeared on me, leaving me in the hands of different creatures who lacked his aliveness, his flexibility of thought.

In New York, my father sat with me in my bedroom as he'd so often done when I was a child and he came to visit. Now he was muted by depression, going through his third divorce. We made a coherent pair, the two of us, both locked into some internal crisis that left us grim and self-involved.

"Let's all take a Vicodin," my father suggested one evening in my bedroom to me and my brother, in an attempt at festivity. I don't remember the rest.

In the spring, a development: a neuroscientist named Oliver Morris now came every Thursday evening to plunge us into a weekly brain tutorial intended as preparation for the following year's curriculum. For three hours at a time, Morris, a rosy-cheeked, boyish academic with impeccable credentials, stood in front of the projection screen, clicking through his slides. GABA. Glutamate. The elemental molecules of brain activity. Inhibitory chemicals. Excitatory chemicals. Click. Click. Click.

UCLA felt like a distant memory. Then, I had thrilled to discover that studying the brain was, in many ways, like studying a brand-new landscape, one whose basic texture was uncanny in its foreignness. There was the hazardous topography—the gyri and sulci—the peaks and valleys of the extraterrestrial-looking wrinkles covering the brain's outer surface. There were the fabulously named structures, which whispered of historical sensibilities: the *hippocampus,* Greek for "sea horse," because that's what it resembles when sliced; the *amygdala,* to denote "almond," the brain's pulsing little nut of a threat detector.

But nothing compared to the aristocratic Nodes of Ranvier, the little gaps along the length of the axon that help the cell's electric message make its precarious passage from one end to the other. *Ranvier, Ranvier:* I pictured some incredible French explorer touching down on this moonscape, having scraped with disaster—wrecked his ship, lost his men—but managing, finally, to find refuge in the Nodes.

And as for the brain's most basic unit, the neuron itself, of which there are billions, each one is endowed at all times with the potential for action, an action which is called, somewhat misleadingly, the "action potential." Will the neuron fire or not fire? That is the question.

Now, seated in the Anna Freud Centre library, where tomes of psychoanalytic classics lined the walls, the neuroscientific material seemed different to me, lodged at an inexplicable remove. *Ranvier, Ranvier, wherefore art thou?* Looking back years later on those hours with Oliver Morris, I better understand the sense of disorientation his lessons induced. The serving up of hard science against the backdrop of Freudian theory was as jarring as it was incomprehensible. It was as if Morris and his particles of GABA and glutamate had blown in from another century and the only thing I could do was bewilderedly gape.

But, as well, I might now argue that feeling alienated by neuroscience was a position implicitly endorsed by many if not most of the psychoanalysts responsible for the bulk of our education. There was, I became aware, a vaguely clandestine atmosphere to this after-hours neuroscience education, delivered when the rest of the building had emptied, the analysts and analysands and analytic candidates all gone home. Neuroscience had little place in our curriculum that year. At all times, it was treated with suspicion by much of the faculty, many of whom were not involved with our unusual master's program and, I was coming to think, did not entirely approve of it. For what could glutamate do towards deepening our understanding of the human psyche? I often heard a version of that question repeated from psychoanalysts resistant to the idea that neuroscientific advances could help further psychological insight. What did the physical properties of the machine have to do with the inner life that arises, somehow, out of it?

2

SEPTEMBER 2007

"Welcome to New Haven," said the man waiting for us with our information packets in hand. "I'm Prakash." It was just after Labor Day at the Yale Child Study Center, our new home base, a red brick building on the edge of the medical school campus. We were here to begin the second half of our two-year education, moving from psychoanalysis to neuroscience. At the moment, on this humid Wednesday, I couldn't begin to imagine how the great unifying process would take place.

At Yale, we had walked into a world of constant, new information, an unending river of small, potentially groundbreaking discoveries, each offering a fresh angle from which to consider the brain. In our Neurobiology of Emotion class, we read about the role of dopamine in monogamy; the neural basis of romantic love; how the amygdala affects long-term memory; how the brain works to help us use thought to regulate strong emotion; how the drug D-cycloserine might be used to treat patients with phobias, restructuring their very memories for the object of dread. All of these were recent studies, published within the last five years, each suggesting the tidal wave of infinite possibility just ahead.

That year, the writer and psychiatrist Norman Doidge was on

the lecture circuit with his new book, *The Brain That Changes Itself.* In it, he explored the idea of "neuroplasticity," the brain's natural capacity to grow new neurons, make new connections between them, and change the degree of influence one neuron might have on another, dialing up or down previously existing connections. Only fifteen years earlier, common wisdom in neuroscience held that brain growth is more or less finished by the age of twenty, that the only changes which occur afterwards are those induced by damage or atrophy. The startlingly recent discovery of "adult neurogenesis," as it is called, was a major breakthrough, a true rethinking of how the brain works. Yet apparently, I was learning, these kinds of paradigm-shifting insights into the functions of the brain were now occurring regularly. Nothing was fixed, nothing impossible.

A page from my notebook:

September 12, 2007/ NEUROIMAGING

The tracer principle: Use a tag or label on a molecule to follow its behavior.

   Decay models:

   Neutron excess—results atoms attempt to return to stable state by emitting neutron deficient positron emissions. The emission produces gamma ray which becomes detectable.

   (Positron encounters electron, they destroy each other, and release a gamma ray.) 180 degrees in orientation (gamma ray).

   However

   Single photon emission tomography (SPECT)/ emitted directly from source, not 2 directional, just one directional. (Thus SPECT is better @ detecting the exact source.)

Our neuroimaging class met once a week. Each Wednesday, a different scientist came to describe his lab's scanning machine of choice. The sheer volume of options amazed me. My days were filled with acronyms. There was the tried and true: the EEG, the hairnet of electrodes that measures only the outermost layer of brain activity, invented in the 1920s and still the preferred tool for many dream researchers. There was MEG, which measured magnetic fields emanating from brain activity; there was SPECT, which could detect patterns of blood flow into tissues and organs. There was PET, which was considered a great step forward when it came out in the 1970s for its ability to look at every part of the brain, not only the outside surface accessible to simpler technology. PET scanners monitor the decay of a radioactive compound, called a tracer, which has been shot into the bloodstream of the person under investigation. But a much more of-the-moment technology in the studies we were busy reading was fMRI, which, like PET, could look at the whole brain at once, but didn't require the use of radioactive materials to do so. And for researchers interested in a different emphasis, there was DTI, or diffusion tensor imaging, which detects activity along the brain's white-matter connections, which is to say axons, the trail of fibers that link every neuron to the next, thereby detailing the relationships between different parts of the brain. The list went on.

As the semester proceeded, it began to dawn on me that the seemingly endless list of options now available for looking at the brain was no mere sideshow: the armament of modern tools is the central fact in explaining the explosion that has taken place in neuroscience over the last two decades. It is technological development that has produced the great boom of energy in the field, the flocks of graduate students filling neuroscience departments.

Walking through campus with my classmates after lecture one day, we struck our over-knowing grad student posture, musing about our perceptions of the great new world of brain scans, deconstructing everything. There was something unsettling about studying all this neurotechnology, a kind of obsession with the machines themselves that seemed at times to obscure the larger purpose, which was, of course, to look at the brain, to better understand the brain. But entrenched as we were in the details of the methods and machines, the brain itself could seem to dip out of view, like the sun sliding down below a gaudy sunset.

In the middle of the first semester, I was on an airplane, watching for a second time a movie called *The Great New Wonderful*. I was waiting for my favorite scene. The movie stars Maggie Gyllenhaal as a cold, trendy New Yorker, a baker of extremely expensive cakes, the kind of cakes that the children of celebrities and hedge fund managers must have at their birthdays and bar mitzvahs. It takes place in the months after 9/11 and shows a group of people who've been set profoundly adrift, but aren't exactly aware of it. It's not very good, I must admit, but something about the movie had hooked into me. I was eager to get to the scene I vividly remembered from when I first saw it, on the long flight from Los Angeles to London that I took when I moved to England for graduate school. In the scene, Gyllenhaal, dressed to perfection, exquisitely burdened, willowy, remote, wanders alone through the massive house of that day's birthday girl, whose cake has been constructed on the theme of "Shakespeare's women." Gyllenhaal is beginning to seem disenchanted with the whole ten-thousand-dollar-cake enterprise, the unthinkable materialism of the life she's staked out for herself. She wanders into a side room, where she finds a group of younger kids taking turns at a karaoke machine. Just as the littlest, chubbiest girl gets up to do her song, someone calls from another room that they're serving the cake now, and the kids all make a mad dash for it, leaving the chubby girl alone at the microphone. But Gyllenhaal leans forward in her chair, gestures to her: *Keep going, I'm here,* waves her hand to say, *I'm listening.* The subtlety of her gesture, the grace of it, had lodged in my memory. I focused in on the screen in front of me. There went the kids to the cake, leaving the little girl standing bereft at the microphone—yet Maggie G. doesn't do anything like what I remember. She makes no gesture at all. She remains completely still in her chair. Somehow she conveys, without moving, without words, the message that I recalled, the message that the girl should go on. And so the girl goes on. She sings: "Your love is better than ice cream, better than anything else that I've tried" . . . It was by far the best scene in the movie. That much remained true. I would think of this moment with Maggie Gyllenhaal again and again: neuroscience had recently shown that even our most vividly drawn memories are nothing if not impermanent.

The name for this particular discovery was still a buzzword in 2007: *memory reconsolidation.* A few days after my encounter with Maggie G., I was back at my desk in Kirtland Hall, in Neurobiology of Emotion class, listening to our soft-spoken professor, Glenn Schafe, telling the story of memory reconsolidation. Schafe slipped it to us in his understated way: he was there when it happened.

Schafe was at New York University, working as a postdoc in the lab of Joseph LeDoux. LeDoux had worked through the 1990s to parse the brain's fear system, delineating, for instance, the role of the amygdala in influencing memories of stressful experiences. In the lab as well was a young postdoc named Karim Nader, who, like Schafe, was there to work towards the lab's central quest of understanding how the brain responds to danger. But in 1996, Nader went to hear a lecture by Eric Kandel, the neuroscientist who would, four years later, be awarded the Nobel Prize. Kandel had spent his long career on the question of how the brain makes new memories. Working on the most granular level, he observed that in order for successful learning to occur in the brain, neurons must instantly manufacture new proteins to make the chemicals flowing between them behave more consequentially. The physical changes that occur are relatively simple, but the implications of Kandel's findings were enormous. New memories restructure the brain in the very moments they are created. Kandel's finding took the concept of learning out of the rarefied cloud of abstraction to which it had always seemed to belong, and placed it for the first time in the ranks of the concrete; learning became, thanks to Kandel, an idea that could be operationalized—an idea, in other words, that could be looked at and measured and talked about specifically.

Based on the work of Kandel and others, the assumption was formed that once an experience has managed to become a memory that has managed to become a long-term memory (outlasting the initial limbo period of seconds or minutes during which so many of our fresh impressions naturally expire), then the information it contains is there to stay; that just as the memory was originally "encoded," so it remains. But listening to Kandel describe his work, Nader had an idea for a new line of inquiry.

Back at the lab, Nader described his plan to LeDoux, who discouraged him from pursuing it, believing it wasn't likely to get results. On an instinct, Nader carried on. He was using the same techniques as Pavlov: he trained four rats by playing a short, high-pitched beep and, directly afterwards, delivering an electrical shock. The education was a quick one: rats need only one training session before they learn to freeze whenever they next hear the same high-pitched beep repeated. But in this version of the experiment, Nader trained the rats, waited a day, replayed the beep, then immediately injected the rats' brains with a drug that blocked the formation of new proteins, including those proteins necessary to the laying down of new memories. If it were true that memories are formed only once—consolidated, as Kandel showed—and stored more or less intact in the brain, then the drug should have no effect on the rats' ability to recall that the beep predicts the electric shock. But if memories are once again labile each time they are recalled, as Nader was beginning to suspect—as uncertain and malleable as if they were brand new—then the drug would be able to distort or even erase the rats' original memory of the meaning of the beep. Which was exactly what Nader found.

By playing the high-pitched beep again but immediately disrupting the proteins required for a memory to first form in the brain, Nader was able to unravel the rats' memories from the previous day. Suddenly, the animals forgot to freeze when they heard their cue. Their Pavlovian conditioning had evaporated. They had no reason to fear an electric shock; they couldn't remember that it was coming.

Nader triumphantly reported his results to LeDoux. He knew it was early days, that there were countless alternative theories and confounding variables he still had to rule out. But he was building a case: he believed it would eventually be possible to show that, on a molecular level, all of our recollections are *always* subject to reinterpretation, editing, and even erasure, porous to the present moment every single time they resurface. Nader believed that far from being static imprints of the original experience, memories are susceptible to alteration the instant they enter our conscious awareness, no matter how long we've stored them—months, years, decades.

So dramatic was the discovery that there was instant push-back, a fact that would become part of Nader's legend. At the Society for Neuroscience Conference in 2001, held that year in San Diego, arguments broke out in conference rooms about the memory reconsolidation hypothesis. Nader would later describe this period as his "shouting phase." He would recall that his mentor, LeDoux, was made "uncomfortable" by the controversy his six-foot-three-inch chain-smoking postdoc was creating. When the moment came for Nader to present his findings, he looked out to a room filled to capacity. "It was the first time they brought out the red ropes at the Society for Neuroscience," he would tell me. There were more than a thousand people in the room, waiting to hear Nader—a young scientist with exactly one published article on memory to his name—explain how it could be that he had made a discovery that ran against the entrenched philosophical assumptions of much of the existing memory research. "I didn't know why this was so controversial. You look at the data, you get the same effects as when you block consolidation. If you're not invested, it's a pretty simple interpretation," Nader would tell me. Nevertheless, he was aware, as he'd later summarize the situation: "I either had a grand slam or this field was going to go down." It was the determining moment. His peers would either walk out of the conference room galvanized, primed to further test and explore Nader's hypotheses, or else they would remain skeptical, unmoved, and not terribly impressed by the thirty-something-year-old scientist responsible for all the undeserved hype. "To make matters worse, a few minutes before my talk, Eric Kandel walks in—and he never comes to these things. He sits down right in front of the podium."

Nader stood up. His voice was shaking as he began, but suddenly he thought: *Just have faith in the experiments.* He ran through his slides, displaying the sizeable amount of data he had by then collected, slides on rat freezing patterns before and after the injection of protein inhibitor and other conditions. "When I sat down, I couldn't believe I was still alive," Nader would tell me. He looked out to see a sea of arms demanding the microphone.

Eric Kandel rose from his chair in the front of the room to signal that he wanted to speak. Kandel's shiny scalp and trademark red bowtie would have been unmistakable to anyone in that room. Kandel turned so that he was partially facing the audience.

"I've been listening very carefully," Nader would remember Kandel saying, "and I think this work is *fabulous.*" Kandel went on to expand upon why. Memory reconsolidation became a viable hypothesis that day.

In the years since, Nader's discovery has helped to redirect how memory is conceived of in neuroscientific labs. Now, people study reconsolidation at Oxford and Harvard and McGill, where Nader has his own lab. The implications of the work are far-reaching. The research has been seized upon, for instance, by the Department of Defense as a potential key to treating post-traumatic stress disorder, the condition afflicting many veterans with vivid flashbacks to traumatic events. If, as Nader's discovery implies, memories are flexible in the moments when they are actively replayed in the mind, then shouldn't it be possible to purposefully modify them? In the case of traumatic memories, to dull the edges? Or eliminate them altogether?

All of which brought me back to turn-of-the-century Vienna. When Sigmund Freud first went to work on his hysterical patients, many of them reported childhood sexual trauma, often at the hands of their own fathers. At first, Freud took them at their word, believing their recollections, but by 1897 he made an abrupt reversal. "I no longer believe in my neurotica," he wrote in a letter to his friend Wilhelm Fliess. The phrase became a part of psychoanalytic history. Freud was now convinced that his patients' stories shouldn't be regarded as facts, necessarily, but rather as fantasies—yet fantasies that were no less relevant to understanding their symptoms than if the sexual encounters they described had indeed occurred. For Freud, what mattered was what his patients *believed* they remembered. It would take neuroscientists a century to back up Freud's perception that memories are fundamentally dynamic.

As in any burgeoning field, by 2007, for every groundbreaking discovery coming out of neuroscience, like, for instance, memory reconsolidation, there was as well a sea of chaff, particularly around the use of brain-scanning technology. In *The New York Times,* I read pieces like "This Is Your Brain on Politics," in which a group of scientists claimed to be able to use brain scanners to detect the political preferences of swing voters. Among other bold statements, the scientists asserted that they could detect the two political candidates least able to engage voters: Barack Obama and John McCain. The very two men who would, of course, later be the presidential nominees, apparently sufficiently engaging. Shortly after their *Times* piece came out, the authors were taken to task for the shortcomings of their study's methods by a second group of neuroscientists, in a scathing letter to the editor. The episode became well known, exposing a rift in the field, a tension around the use of still-new technology for experiments that were full of popular appeal, but notably low on rigor.

Suddenly, there was a claim being made, a flag planted: neuroscientific findings were morphing into our cultural truths. Everywhere I looked it seemed that we were being defined by what our brains were doing. We were "hardwired." We were a collection of parts, of "circuits" and "networks" that "light up" when "activated." Everywhere, there were hucksters and geniuses, all trying to colonize the new world of the brain.

At the Yale bookstore, a towering pile of *Proust Was a Neuroscientist* held pride of place for weeks. The cover was alluring: a madeleine floating on a pale blue background. It was the debut book by the writer Jonah Lehrer, who over the next five years would frequently write in grandiloquent terms about how neuroscience had solved some of the greatest mysteries of human life. With his pleasingly accessible prose, he would dispel the opacity around how we make decisions, and then, in his third book, he would tackle the creative process, explaining in *Imagine: How Creativity Works* that the moment of artistic breakthrough can be understood, in part, as "alpha waves emanating from the right hemisphere." Lehrer's prolific writing seemed to answer an intense popular craving to see the mind's most private machinations laid out in simple and definitive neuroscientific terms. I was often confused by Lehrer's confident assertions as he described the science that supposedly illuminated all of these great unknowns. I was missing something, I believed.

. . .

News from New York; my father called to report the following event: "I was pouring my coffee this morning, and suddenly, I felt some hope." He had received a letter a few months before from a listener to his radio program, inquiring after an obscure piece of Frank Sinatra arcana, one of my father's specialties. He recognized her name at once—Zohra Lampert had been a distinguished theater actress in the 1960s, and part of the whole John Cassavetes scene, the movie director for whom "authenticity" was utmost: the obsession with, the search for, the stripped-down truth at the center of everything. Zohra's enduring legacy could perhaps be traced to her role in *Splendor in the Grass,* as the pizza waitress with whom Warren Beatty finally runs off.

It turned out that Zohra now lived just down the street from my father. This boded well, as in his current state of mind and body, he was unable to travel much farther. He took me to meet Zohra one weekend when I came in from school. Her apartment looked like a set from a movie about a New York intellectual living minimally. She had almost no furniture. What she had were books, mostly by the towering German philosophers of the eighteenth century, and in particular Hegel, to whom she had devoted a great deal of the last two decades. Sweetly, she tried to make a bond with me by telling me how much she admired the work of Sigmund Freud. "Oh really?" I said. "I've fallen quite out of love with him." Silence descended in her spare living room. I didn't even know why I had rebuffed her gesture of friendship. I still cared about Freud, though the relationship had become more complicated since spending time with his descendants in London. But as my father and I left Zohra's apartment, I couldn't help but notice that a certain buoyancy had returned to his demeanor.

.   .   .

That January, I spent much of a bitterly cold Martin Luther King Day weekend on Park Avenue, at the Waldorf Astoria Hotel, attending the annual meeting of the American Psychoanalytic Association, arguably the most lustrous and powerful of such institutions. "Predictions of our demise are premature!" I heard one psychoanalyst declare to another, standing in the ornate marble lobby. For the next three days, we would be hearing about such familiar analytic staples as masturbation fantasies and masculinity, but also on the schedule were sessions addressed to the possibility of linking psychoanalysis and neuroscience. By now, it was the inevitable conversation.

Up in the cushy Sutton Suite on the first afternoon, a crowd of forty or so gathered around a long table for a workshop called "What Does Dostoevsky Teach Us About Psychoanalysis?" Presiding over the discussion were the psychoanalysts Paul and Anna Ornstein, Hungarian émigrés, husband and wife. Outside, the sun passed behind a cloud, and the room settled in. People took out their Dostoevskys.

"Freud thought *The Brothers Karamazov* was in the same league as *Oedipus Rex* and *Hamlet*," Paul Ornstein began. "He thought that all three of these works of literature dealt with the Oedipus complex, essentially."

Ornstein emphasized Dostoevsky's ability to access his inner world in order to create complex characters. He could do this, Ornstein repeatedly observed, even though he was writing "prior to Freud." Ornstein wanted to know, what did everyone think this book was about?

"The central conflict is between freedom and the wish to submit," one female analyst said. "Each character is dealing with the unconscious wish to say: force me to believe, force me to give myself up to you."

Another hand sprouted up.

"There is an opinion over there," Anna Ornstein said, pointing.

"A sense of seeking the object," said a woman with a Russian accent. "The murder of the father made me think the father is the embodiment of grabbing that object and eating that object and consuming that object and inciting the envy and the same appetites in the children who are already so very hungry for the object." She gestured wildly with her hands.

It was one more encounter with that particular psychoanalytic *way:* the unabashed passion, the fever of engagement. In the popular imagination, psychoanalysis conjures up silent doctors in dimly lit rooms, witnesses to the unfurling of dream images and childhood memories. And couches, lots of couches, and lots of time spent lying on them. Expensive time. This is the stereotype, the myth, but what is true is that the psychoanalytic project—a thoroughgoing and uninhibited exploration of one's unconscious mind—might or might not be able to survive in its current form. An analysis can go on for years. Until recently, there has been relatively little empirical proof that it works. Up against the quick and easy fixes of prescription medication or short-term, practically oriented cognitive behavioral therapy—and under the skeptical eye of insurance companies—the field of psychoanalysis has taken on the aspect of the underdog. At the Waldorf Astoria, the implicit question was being asked yet again: Where do we go from here?

There were, in a sense, some responses on offer to that very question. There was the surprisingly titled "Psychoanalysis in China" workshop, which revealed a burgeoning interest in psychoanalysis among the new Chinese middle and upper classes. Several psychoanalysts at the meeting had treated Chinese patients and described cultural differences they'd encountered. The fact that Eastern cultures regard identity as interdependent, as part of a family unit, for example, clouds the psychoanalytic focus on the "separation-individuation" phase of development. Likewise, in China it is common for children to sleep in the same room or even bed with their parents for years—which means that Chinese children often have multiple exposures to the "primal scene" of parental intercourse that Freud regarded as a universal childhood trauma. How to deal with these differences? How to assimilate Eastern values into a fundamentally Western treatment philosophy? There weren't necessarily answers here, but, as usual, there were questions. Grant writers and supervisors were urgently needed, it was announced, and so were those willing to analyze a Chinese patient on Skype. Yellow cards were distributed for people to sign up. The room was galvanized.

Nowhere was the divide between classic and modern, old and new, more apparent than at the conference "poster session"—a scientific tradition, not a psychoanalytic one, where researchers show off their latest work, each poster documenting the nuts and bolts of the experimental process, its methods and results, its *who what when where how.* Fifteen or so small teams displayed posters explaining their current studies. Several involved the use of brain imaging technology, a reflection of the pressure that many in the field now felt to substantiate psychoanalytic theories with empirical evidence. There was, for instance, "MRI Brain Changes in Psychoanalysis," a study that was being conducted by the research psychiatrist Andrew Gerber and his team at Columbia. Using brain imaging, they were trying to identify the neural changes that result from a year in psychoanalytic treatment.

From the University of Ghent came another study, "Anal and

Oral Word Use in Relation to Dependency and Self-Criticism."
Standing in front of the display, Stijn Vanheule, a young Dutch
PhD, proudly pointed to his results: people classified as "dependent" are significantly more likely to use "oral" words, such as
mouth, breast, and *eating.* In comparison to the images of brain activation ten feet away, Dr. Vanheule's Freudian investigation seemed
particularly retro. But also, in a sense, particularly welcome.

Back at school, as the winter wore on, I was soon fully launched
on my dissertation research. Based on the archive of files at the
Yale Trauma Clinic where I worked, I was writing about "intergenerational trauma patterns" in families. In my apartment, piles of
studies about the effects of stress on the brain were stacked on the
floor. Except for the work of the more prominent neuroscientists
of our time—such as Antonio Damasio, Eric Kandel, and Joseph
LeDoux—I tended not to focus on research conducted before the
year 2000. It was a prejudice I picked up by example, observing the
habits of graduate students around me. Neuroscience was whizzing
along at such a pace that research conducted only ten years earlier
had likely been improved upon since. Even if it hadn't, its date alone
cast a pall of obsolescence.

On weekends, I hunkered down in the basement of the medical
school library, lacing lines of neon pink and orange through pages
of scientific text. I noticed that I was beginning to gain a certain
degree of fluency in this new language, suddenly able to understand
sentences like: "Whether anxiety disorders stem from too much
'bottom-up' amygdala activation or too little 'top-down' inhibitory
control, facilitation of mPFC activity might be effective in control-
ling an overactive amygdala."

But something else: it continued to be true that in much of the neuroscientific research I was looking at, the mind as I knew it—in all of its quirky, complicated familiarity—was rarely in evidence. One particular experiment stays with me years later. Imagine the following. You are twenty, a sophomore in college. You're majoring in psychology, which requires you to volunteer for at least three studies in the psychology department every semester. Or maybe you're doing it for the fifteen dollars they give out at the end. You see a flier. You go into the lab and a little drove of grad students descends upon you, purposeful, focusing in, giving you your instructions. They warn you to take off every bit of metal you have on your person before you go into the MRI room, because the magnet is so powerful that even a bobby pin becomes a flying weapon in its vicinity, hurtling at warp speed through the air, capable of blinding someone. You're beginning to regret your decision to come here today. You can't remember if you have metal fillings. If you move your head at all once you're in the machine, they say, it will render the data meaningless. We'll have to start from scratch. You cannot move your head. Not at all. Not one inch. Are you clear on this point? You put on the headphones they give you and lie down. Your head is immobilized in Styrofoam, your neck is stiff, and now the narrow tray you're lying on is sliding backwards, like a mechanical tongue retracting into its robot mouth. You take a foot-long journey and then you reach your destination. You're looking up at a small television screen, deep in the depths of this smooth tin igloo. You are aware of your legs and feet, splayed out on view for the grad students watching through the glass window.

The machine, operating at full tilt, clanks and thuds, much more loudly than you would have expected. No whispery iPhone magic in these parts. On the contrary: it sounds like there are small children somewhere inside, throwing tantrums with pots and pans. You're not having a particularly good time. You contemplate squeezing the ball they've given you to hold, which you've been told will alert them to your distress, the fMRI version of a panic button. But then the screen above your face flickers on and you're shown seven minutes of *Bambi*. You're grateful to be watching something familiar, even though what they're showing you is the scene where Bambi's mother dies. Of course. What else? The *Bambi* clip ends. The screen fades to black. A voice pipes into your ear. Please state your mood on a scale of one to nine. Well, you know what to do. It's not subtle, what they're asking here. And you don't want to accidentally score like a sociopath. No. You might date that intense little grad student later, for all you know. Duly, you report that your mood is "slightly sad" or even, for good measure, "significantly sad." You hope they'll let you go home now.

This is a version of the scenario you might endure if you were one of the volunteers who came into the lab at Duke University to participate in the experiment being conducted there, the experiment that would culminate in a prestigious paper, published in the journal *Biological Psychiatry* in 2006, titled: "Mood Alters Amygdala Activation to Sad Distractors During an Attentional Task."

I read this study while hunched in my usual position in the library of the medical school. The experiment was conducted by three researchers named Lihong Wang, Kevin LaBar, and Greg McCarthy. They wanted to investigate whether depression affects what we pay attention to and how we pay attention to it. In the largest sense, they were exploring the question of how depression causes people to filter the world around them in such a way as to reinforce their state of mind, selecting out the moments that would contradict their mood in favor of those that confirm it.

The authors had set themselves the tricky task of inducing "depression" in their subjects—or, at least, a laboratory-produced model of depression, which is to say a temporary state of sadness.

I proceeded to the heart of the study's methods section. How, I wondered, were these three researchers going to manufacture depression? Like many studies of this kind, the researchers excluded subjects who had, or had ever had, depression in real life. Too complicating. Much more clean and controlled to avoid actual depression while studying depression. Instead, twenty subjects were selected "with no self-reported history of neurological or psychiatric illness or drug addiction." (I tried to imagine the most cheerful cohort I possibly could. The Duke Glee Club?) How would Wang, LaBar, and McCarthy manage to pull off an effective "mood induction" at exactly the expedient moment, while the subjects were lying in the scanner, just before they were given the experimental task? Moods, as many of us know from experience, are not often susceptible to this kind of domestication. On the contrary, they go where they want, when they want.

The authors acknowledged the challenge they faced. "Fewer neuroimaging studies have examined mood induction in healthy adults," they wrote in their introduction, noting that the various techniques that had been used for such a thing had shown "variable results." Their solution: sad movie clips. The reader was assured that all the footage used in this study (from *Bambi, Terms of Endearment, Titanic,* and *I Love Lucy*—the latter, one assumes, for the purpose of a comparison trial) had been "rated sequentially on a 9-point Likert-type scale for each of sixteen emotion terms to evaluate their affective properties. The sixteen items consisted of the following emotions: amusement, anger, arousal, confusion, contempt, contentment, disgust, embarrassment, fear, happiness, interest, pain, relief, sadness, surprise and tension. Only those movies that were rated high on sadness and pain and low on other emotions were selected for the sad mood induction."

Once the subjects had been shown the designated movie clips and their sad mood presumably induced (and the researchers had confirmed the efficacy of their sad-mood induction technique not with the study's actual participants, but with a previous group of volunteers who had been brought into the lab solely for the purpose of figuring out whether the movies actually produced sad moods, as assessed on a mood measurement scale), they then proceeded to the "emotional oddball task." On the screen where *Bambi* had recently concluded, subjects were now told to focus on a visual target—circles—that would pop up in a stream of rectangles. In the midst of these circles and rectangles, the authors explain, "distracting sad and neutral scenes were intermittently presented."

What the authors wanted to determine was whether these sad images, when presented to subjects who were in a sad mood, took on a heightened salience, enough to hijack the subject's attention from the task at hand, which was to notice the circles appearing among the rectangles. I was curious to discover what sad images Wang, LaBar, and McCarthy had decided to show their twenty volunteers. One, I discovered, was a photo of a woman crying into a telephone. The pictures all came from online stock photos and were selected for their depictions of "humans crying or portraying sad facial expression," or "scenes of despair, grief, internment, incarceration, and poverty."

Later, I would learn sophisticated critiques of brain-scanning studies, critiques having to do with the blurry assumptions researchers make about where in an individual brain the amygdala even is (it differs for everybody), and how to decide which statistical analyses to run (with countless options, each one offering a different spin on the data). I would come to understand that there was already a vigorous debate within the field itself over the value of fMRI studies, neuroscientists arguing with one another about whether these measurements were valid at all, and if so, to what extent. I would hear critiques based on Bayesian analyses, on voxel placement, on designated p-values. All later. Then, sitting in the medical school library amid piles of studies on the traumatized brain, grappling with the scientific literature that was still new to me, what I thought about was how dramatically the richness of Freud's ideas crashed and burned at the doors to the fMRI lab. Sadness was what happened to you after you watched *Bambi*. Mood was your score on the Beck Depression Inventory. Scores < 9 = not depressed. I was struck by the thought that Freud's "Mourning and Melancholia," a text written nearly a century earlier, could seem to powerfully illuminate a dynamic at the very heart of the opaque affliction that had plagued my father and so many others—while a cutting-edge, neuroscientific work could be constructed around such a simplified version of "depression" that I had to wonder what it was I was actually learning when I read the authors' conclusion that their subjects' ability to spot circles amid rectangles was somewhat slowed down by the appearance of sad images in the wake of sad movie clips—and that the amygdala was involved.

In truth, I was focused on Wang and co's study not because it stuck out in any way from the vast quantity of research pouring out of neuroimaging labs but rather because it didn't. What it shared in common with other study designs I'd encountered was, among other things, an apparent lack of clinical perspective. For instance, to address the very premise of the experiment: sadness is not the same thing as depression. They are not interchangeable concepts. A psychologist or psychiatrist or psychoanalyst, with experience in treating an actual patient, would be likely to remark immediately on this most basic aspect of the study's approach. Wang and his coauthors do not claim otherwise, yet they gloss over the distinction, and they certainly don't probe for what's informative or interesting about the differences. If a participant can check the right number on a mood measurement scale, the study's rationale goes, that participant's brain activity can tell us something about depression.

In the logic of many experiments I encountered, I feared that human emotions were being reduced to cartoon versions of themselves. Each was simple, discrete, and readily identifiable. *Sad* was different from *angry,* which was different from *ashamed.* There was no blurring of boundaries between them, no complexity, no mess. For the sake of science, each emotion under scrutiny must be lifted as if with sterile tweezers out of the human heart and slid beneath the microscope. Nowhere did I find an acknowledgment that these formulations did not actually resemble human experience; that they were, at best, radically impoverished sketches of inner life.

In the early 1960s, long before I got to New Haven, it was Yale researchers who had carried out perhaps the most notorious social psychology study of all: Milgram's Experiment. Dressed in white lab coats, the researchers instructed their volunteers to press a button that, they were told, delivered an electric shock to a person in the next room, visible through a glass window, every time that person made an error repeating back the list of word-pairs he was supposed to be memorizing. The volunteers didn't know that the recipients of the electric shocks were in fact "confederates"—researchers in disguise—and the shocks weren't real. The confederates would writhe convincingly in pain at each press of the button. After a few rounds, the volunteers would usually begin to protest. *Are you sure, doctor? Are you sure this is okay?* And each time, the man in the white lab coat would tell them: "Continue please. The experiment requires that you continue. It is absolutely essential that you continue. You have no other choice, you must go on."

Stanley Milgram had designed the study as an investigation into the horrors of World War II. He ran it many times, with different groups of volunteers, and he saw that most were willing to follow instructions and deliver steadily accelerating doses of electric shocks to the person rigged up to the machine, even as that person appeared to be suffering more and more acutely. From these observations, Milgram drew a Hannah Arendt–like conclusion: evildoing was nothing special. It was dormant everywhere, just waiting for the right circumstances to ignite, the right authority figure to come along and deliver his sinister instructions.

But I sympathized with Milgram's volunteers. I was finding it difficult—exceedingly difficult—to take ownership of doubt when that doubt stood opposed to the white coats of science. Who was I to protest scientific authority?

Late that winter, an e-mail circulated around our little group. It was from Judit, our eldest member, she of the jet-black curls and bright red lipstick, a practicing psychiatrist in Budapest before she'd come back to school to get another degree.

Subject: Meeting M Solms
hey guys, again. so Mark Solms is happy to meet all of
us on febr 2nd in nyc. Would be great if we all could meet him—
I think
this is an exceptional opportunity. if this date is
not good for everyone, we should find another one.
i know i sound very
official but please let me know asap xx

I knew Mark Solms's name. We all did. He had a huge reputation within the particular neuroscientific territory that we, the psychoanalytically inclined, inhabited. He was a psychoanalyst, neuropsychologist, Freud translator, and dream researcher, but, most relevant to our purposes, he was the public face of the effort to launch the new, interdisciplinary undertaking that he himself had named neuropsychoanalysis.

Dear Judit,

Thanks. Mark says he will meet you all (how many of you
are there?) at the New York Psychoanalytic Institute at
1:00 pm
On that Saturday (February 2).
The meeting will probably take place in the Board Room.

Cordially,
Paula

Solms lived in Cape Town but came to New York every month for different engagements, including a lecture series he had run since the early 1990s, inviting neuroscientists of every stripe to speak about their work—on topics like memory, emotion, and unconscious cognition—to audiences of psychoanalysts. The lecture series was one of the countless tactics Solms had implemented over the years in his effort to effect the integration he envisioned.

We were supposed to meet Solms at the end of one of these lectures, but when we arrived at the New York Psychoanalytic Society & Institute, a boxy, gray building on East Eighty-Second Street, we found the heavy wooden door locked and no sign of anyone inside. We knocked. We waited. We knocked. Finally, the door opened. A short man with a bad leg, a foreign accent, and a feather duster in one hand peered out at us discouragingly.

"Dr. Solms has left the building," he said, and began to close the door.

Suddenly, a man in a flapping trench coat joined us on the sidewalk.

"The Yalies!" he said, leaning in.

I recognized him as Dr. David Goldman, Upper East Side psychoanalyst, whom I'd met at a conference the month before.

"Mark Solms was looking for you, but he left because he thought you weren't coming," he said.

We asked where he went. We asked the custodian, still in his territorial stance in the doorway, whether he knew how we might reach Dr. Solms.

"He's gone," the man said, with Eastern European finality.

"Does he have a cell phone? Will he be back?" we asked.

"No," he said, and successfully closed the door.

Dr. Goldman, it seemed, had now joined our cause. He pulled his digital camera from around his neck and began to show us pictures of Solms that he'd taken that morning, at the lecture we hadn't attended. We clustered together to look at Dr. Goldman's viewfinder. Mark Solms had a large, expressive face, a prominent, rounded nose. I looked up from the camera. Where would a famous neuropsychoanalyst go after being ditched by a group of grad students he had graciously agreed to meet with? The answer seemed clear: to lunch. From where we were standing, I could see a row of restaurants on the perpendicular avenue. One little trattoria stood out somehow, for the crisp white lettering on its canopy. On impulse, I jogged down Eighty-Second Street, across the avenue, and into the restaurant. It was quiet inside and empty, except for a group of about six or so sitting around a table in the front. There, unmistakably, presiding over the conversation, was Mark Solms.

I felt ridiculous as I interrupted the group.

"Excuse me, but are you Mark Solms?"

"Yes," he said, unsurprised to be recognized by someone he'd never met before.

I explained who I was and apologized for the confusion. We'd planned to meet him at the end of the lecture, I said; we'd heard the speaker before, and decided not to come early to hear her again.

"I can't say I blame you," he told me, his British-inflected South African accent warm and commanding. We agreed to regroup in an hour. The thin blond woman sitting next to him, her chair drawn in close, didn't look happy to hear this. Solms was one of those people, it was immediately clear, whose departure precipitates the end of the party.

· · ·

An hour later, we took our seats around a heavy wooden table in a damp room on the top floor of the institute. The room was bare except for the requisite images of Freud—in this case, a ceramic bust on the mantelpiece and a photograph, hanging crooked on the wall, of Freud, head swiveled, looking straight into the camera. I thought of this as his feline shot. If I became an expert on anything in graduate school, it was the Sigmund Freud iconography that psychoanalytic institutes across the world invariably display, sometimes reverentially, always superstitiously. Like many of these institutes, the New York chapter felt as if no one had been inside since the 1970s. It was hushed and musty and intermittently lit. Paint peeled. You traveled from the bottom to the top in a tiny wood-paneled elevator, the kind you operate manually, pushing a lever to steer.

Solms was tall and solid, thick-wristed, big-headed. His skin was ruddy and dented in places; there was, in the relation of his arms to his torso to his neck, something distinctly simian, a raw, primitive quality that made you think about evolution. He was in his late forties but looked older, as if he'd been too extravagant with his stash of vitality. His gray hair, poking up in all directions, was completely unattended to, like a member of the family with whom he was no longer on speaking terms.

"Well, I'll just talk," Solms said. "Then you can tell me, that's not what we want. I say again, I'm thrilled to meet you. I was very worried about how on earth they were going to teach this course. There aren't many people in the field who truly have integrated psychoanalysis and neuroscience. It sounds like a little bit of this, a little bit of that, a little bit of trying to cobble together things where you're going to have to do the work of actually making the connections—and it's fucking impossible that you're expected to do that!"

At that, my classmates and I lost it. We were laughing uproariously. We were throwing our heads back. It was as if a year and a half of academic ambiguity had been cleared away with one profanity.

"I started working in this area in the mid 1980s and I've been trying to persuade colleagues on both sides that this is a good thing to do ever since. It's been a hell of a journey. I've had many disappointments along the way. It's not been as easy as I would have thought it would be to get psychoanalysts to see the necessity of using what you learn from the point of view of the neurosciences about the mind. It *must* be relevant to what they do, just because there can only be one mind. There can't be a mind for neuroscience and a mind for psychoanalysis. There's only one human mind."

Could this have really been the first time I'd considered the problem with such crisp simplicity? In one swoop, Solms had tied up the threads of uncertainty I'd been tugging along for the last eighteen months. In the jumble of subjects we had thus far encountered, from countertransference to tracer principle, from mind to machine, there was precious little cohesion, even though, as Solms reminded us, psychoanalysis and neuroscience were talking about the same thing. Psychoanalysis was looking at the brain from the inside out: what does it feel like to *be* this thing? Neuroscience was looking at the brain from the outside in, measuring its behavior, investigating its physical mechanisms. They were two views of one object. There could be only one mind. To hear Solms put it in these stripped-down terms felt like hearing it for the first time.

Solms had first trained in neuropsychology, he told us, a branch of neurology that draws links between people's external behaviors and the specific regions of the brain involved in producing them. Solms went into the field thinking that, of all the subsets of neuroscience, neuropsychology was, as he put it, "where you're most likely to find out about the person himself." But he was disappointed. Neuropsychology seemed to avoid everything that had to do with questions of personality, emotion, motivation—in other words, the things we mean when we speak of "human nature." Instead, the operating gaze was trained onto the strictly quantifiable: How many digits could the patient hold in his working memory? Neuropsychology, Solms discovered, asked black-and-white questions that could be answered on standardized tests.

"Oliver Sacks has this saying: neuropsychology is admirable, but it excludes the psyche," Solms said. Around the table, our group nodded in unison. We could relate to the sentiment. Motivated by what he experienced as the shortcomings of his profession, Solms moved to London in his late twenties and began to train as a psychoanalyst. For years, he lived a double life, working with brain-damaged patients by day at the Royal London Hospital, training at the Institute of Psychoanalysis by night.

"Freud's intention was never to have only one perspective, only one method," Solms said. "Even at the beginning of psychoanalysis, Freud took what he could from every discipline to try and cobble together a theory of how this might tick. He developed a pure psychology knowing that one day it would be possible to supplement and correct it with neuroscientific methods. He said that repeatedly."

Solms carried on in his parallel careers, he told us, treating patients with brain damage who came into the neurosurgery ward at the Royal London, immersing himself in his psychoanalytic education in the evening. Despite the schism that had opened up between them, psychoanalysis and neuroscience were, to Solms, intuitively compatible. He did not at first understand that this belief, this inclination, would be seen by many as controversial or problematic. What he saw was that his psychoanalytic training gave him a new layer of clarity, filling in gaps in his understanding that he hadn't even known were there, recasting his perspective on the brain-damaged patients he treated every day in the neurosurgery ward.

It became clear to Solms that it was only with the help of thinking from the point of view of the mind that he could begin to understand the brain.

"I say it was obvious to me—why wasn't it obvious to everyone?" Solms said. "Like everything else, it was personal. My brother was brain-injured. When he was six, he fell off the roof and suffered a closed head injury. I saw that my brother is not who he was. His personality is different and our whole family is different. All of that because this organ is not functioning as it was before."

It struck me, listening to Solms, that this felt like intimacy. It felt like intimacy despite my sense that this was a story Solms often told. It clinched some warming suspicion in me that this person was an interesting *character*. The word appeared in my head unbidden.

There was a pause in the conversation. We looked up to see that the last of the wintry daylight had started to fade. Somehow, two hours had passed.

"If you seriously want to give your life to working on this, I'll do anything I can to help you," Solms said, speaking quickly, wrapping up, extending a flurry of encouraging words and generous offers.

We must all be in touch and let him know. He would be in New York on the first weekend of every month, like always.

"I live in Cape Town for reasons that have to do with the rest of my life," he said, as he stood up to leave. It was like Brigadoon, receding into the mist. And then he was gone, down the rickety elevator and out the door.

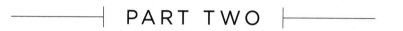

PART TWO

3

BY JUNE 2008, I had finished graduate school, turned in my the-
sis on "intergenerational patterns of trauma," packed up my New
Haven apartment, and was preparing to move into a red barn in
a field in New Hampshire. But I knew I wasn't finished with the
neuropsychoanalytic universe. It had been four months since I'd
met him and still, I was curious about Mark Solms. The time my
classmates and I had spent in his company had been, for reasons
both explicable and not, a rare spot of vibrancy. I had not seen him
since.

This was how I found myself sitting in a lecture hall in the
Montreal Neurological Institute one hot weekend in July. I had
come to attend the conference that Solms hosted in a different
city every year, the annual meeting of the International Neuropsychoanalysis Society, of which Solms was founder and president. Over the next three days, we would be hearing about such
topics as "The Neuropsychoanalysis of Psychological Defense in
the Neurological Patient" and "What the Human Face Tells the
Human Brain About Conflict." Gathered together were shrinks of
all kinds: psychiatrists, psychologists, psychoanalysts, and social
workers. There were brain people too: neuropsychologists, neuroscientists, neurosurgeons. There were lab assistants and PhD students, and there was one man in the back who was conspicuously

out of his mind, dropping his pencil into the aisle every ten minutes or so and rising, unsteadily, to retrieve it. Outside the auditorium, patients were going by in wheelchairs, or standing around in bathrobes with strange caps on their heads, a hundred colorful wires attached to their skulls. This had become my milieu.

The day's schedule announced Dr. Suzanne Corkin, a neuropsychologist at MIT. There is invariably one reason why Corkin is invited anywhere, and that reason is the most famous patient in neurological history, the patient known as H.M.

And who hasn't heard about H.M.? He has fueled a veritable industry of scientific research, think pieces, biographies, dramatic adaptions, and memoirs.

Henry Molaison (as his 2008 obituary revealed him publicly for the first time) was a man from Connecticut with severe epilepsy. From boyhood, he'd had near-daily seizures, causing him to drop out of high school, unable to finish until the age of twenty-one. The drugs he was given failed to contain his condition. Finally, in 1953, the surgeon William Scoville, in Hartford, Connecticut, decided H.M. was a candidate for what Scoville would later term "a frankly experimental procedure."

Scoville was one of many American doctors who believed in psychosurgery: removing or disconnecting whole brain regions in order to address psychiatric irregularities. Since the 1930s, surgery had been considered a promising treatment course for thousands of these patients—most famously, perhaps, Rosemary Kennedy, admitted by her father, Joseph Kennedy, when she was twenty-three years old, for being difficult, "moody," and likely sexually promiscuous. A surgeon named Watts used an instrument that could have doubled as a butter knife to destroy major swaths of her frontal lobes. She lived the rest of her life in a Wisconsin convent, dependent on the care of the nuns. (Women were twice as likely as men to wind up on the operating table for brain alterations.)

Though their problem was not psychiatric, epileptics were seen as good candidates for surgery because of the nature of their disorder: too much electrical activity emanating from discrete focal points of the brain. At Hartford Hospital, Scoville tried twice to pinpoint the locus of H.M.'s seizure activity. He wasn't able to. But he did know that the activity likely originated in the temporal lobes, the area of the brain just behind our ears. On the day of the operation, Scoville drilled through H.M.'s temples and, inserting his tiny vacuum first on the left side, then on the right, sucked out most of H.M.'s hippocampus and amygdala, along with portions of the cortex. H.M. was conscious the whole time, since the brain doesn't have pain receptors. But he wouldn't be able to remember the surgery.

In fact, he wouldn't be able to consciously remember anything new at all from 1953 until his death more than fifty years later. What Scoville hadn't understood, what no one had understood, was that the hippocampus is the seat of memory formation in the brain. The situation was as it had been with language a century before: no one had connected speech to any one specific location in the brain until 1861 when the neurologist Paul Broca performed the autopsy on his former patient Monsieur Leborgne. Until Scoville had vacuumed up both of H.M.'s hippocampi, neurologists hadn't imagined that memory could be somehow tucked away in these seahorse-shaped structures, which occupy mere centimeters of the neural landscape. Yet H.M.'s radical amnesia was immediately apparent. He didn't know where he was or why. He couldn't find his way to the bathroom even after repeated trips. When his parents had brought him to the hospital, they had felt that the burden of his seizures was too great for any of them to continue to bear. Now they had on their hands a man who couldn't remember his own age, or what he'd eaten for breakfast, or even whether he had eaten breakfast. H.M. could remember events from his past before the surgery, though his memory for them was flattened, lacking the rich texture of details infused with emotion that define our sense of our own histories. But he knew the basic facts of his life up until 1953. What he could no longer manage was new, declarative memory, which is to say, any memory that can be consciously described: what movie you saw yesterday afternoon, where you were on 9/11, what your father's face looked like as the Red Sox finally won a World Series—the infinity of tiny plot points we can command at any moment to remind ourselves of who we are. What made H.M.'s case so unusual—and scientifically invaluable—was that although his capacity to form new memories was gone, his intellect remained undiminished. H.M.'s amnesia, produced with surgical precision, was "pure." He became the dictionary definition of amnesiac, the yardstick against which all other cases were measured. For the next decades, in the scientific literature, cases of amnesia were described as being "as bad as H.M." or "not as bad as H.M."

The case of H.M. was a tragedy for the Molaison family and a breakthrough for neuroscience, one that has arguably illuminated more about the nature of memory than any single patient, study, or experiment before or since. Until H.M. emerged from the operating room in 1953 and asked his parents and doctors where he was and what he was doing there, scientists didn't know that the hippocampus is the essential brain region for memory. In the decades to come, H.M., the ever compliant research subject, demonstrated by his performance on every imaginable neuropsychological test that the brain has multiple memory systems—short-term, long-term, procedural, declarative—and that different kinds of memories are stored in different parts. H.M. could no longer say offhand whether he was young or old, whether his parents were dead, or how he knew Suzanne Corkin, who became his de facto scientific guardian, leading the research on his case. Yet when he looked in the mirror, he wasn't stunned to see a white-haired man with a big belly and wrinkles on his face looking back at him. Only minutes before, he would have told his interviewer that he was a young man, and still the aged reflection in the mirror always struck him as somehow recognizable. H.M., who has been described as cheerful, docile, and witty by those who knew him, would just shrug and say, "Well, I'm not a boy." Similarly, he would be stunned and distraught each time he was told of his father's death, from emphysema, when H.M. was forty. Yet, about four years after his father had died, H.M. turned to one of his doctors and, mentioning his father, said: "You see, I am not easy in my mind. On the one side I think he has been called—he's gone—but on the other I think he's alive." H.M. was shaking. "I can't figure it out." As for Suzanne Corkin herself, whose face he looked at probably more than one thousand times in the forty years she devoted to studying him in her lab at MIT, well, he believed they had met at East Hartford High School. H.M. retained a sense of the familiar even in the absence of certainty. This alone was a novel and illuminating detail of how memory works in the brain.

And scientists also discovered that H.M. could still learn certain types of new information—what is now known as procedural memory—the "how to" information that we all know without being able to explicitly spell it all out, like how to drive a car, ride a bike, or tie our shoelaces. These are skills we have at our command; they are memories, but implicit ones. H.M. was able to master such tricks as sketching the outline of a star on a piece of paper, while able to watch his progress only in a mirror, a test known as the "mirror star task." It's notoriously difficult to do, and yet, on each consecutive day that he was asked to do it, even without remembering that he had done it the day before, his mastery expanded significantly. Thus, scientists understood that procedural memory must not rely on the hippocampus. Indeed, H.M.'s case launched thousands of studies of the hippocampus, each one trying to understand more and more specifically the way memories are formed and stored and then remembered, or, in the language of brain science, "retrieved."

After H.M., "everyone wanted their own amnesiac," observed the legendary neuropsychologist Brenda Milner, who wrote the first groundbreaking papers on H.M. in the 1950s. H.M., neuroscience's accidental celebrity, conferred huge renown upon the handful of doctors involved in his care. Suzanne Corkin was foremost among them. Now, taking her place up on the stage of the Montreal Neurological Institute, Corkin looked to be in her sixties, her brown hair short and professional. In keeping with the official theme of the conference, she was going to be addressing the question of whether or not H.M. had "a sense of self."

When Corkin put on a tape recording of an interview she had conducted with H.M. only a few years before, everyone leaned in, rapt by the sound of his voice, the famous textbook case come alive.

"When you're not at MIT, what do you do during a typical day?" she began.

"I don't remember," H.M. said on the recording, sounding cheerful and befuddled and old.

"Do you know what you did yesterday?"

"No, I don't."

"How about this morning?"

"I don't even remember that."

"Could you tell me what you had for lunch today?"

"No, to tell you the truth."

"What do you think you'll do tomorrow?"

"Whatever's beneficial."

"Good answer," Corkin assured the cooperative patient. She continued: "I wanted to ask you some questions about World War II. Remember World War II?"

"Yeah."

"When was World War II?"

"Well, we entered it on the seventh of December."

"Of what year?"

"Nineteen thir—nineteen *forty*."

"Hm. Now, who were we at war with?"

"Well, the Nazis, in a way," said H.M.

"Can you tell me who the world leaders were during that time? Their names?"

"Well . . . the president being Roosevelt."

"Hm. What was his first name?"

A pause.

"Oh dear, I have an argument with myself because he had an uncle, or someone earlier in his family that had been our president too."

"Exactly."

"Franklin," H.M. said, after another moment's consideration.

"Good for you. What was his middle name?"

"Delano."

"Good. Perfect. Who's the president of the United States now?"

"That I couldn't tell you. That I don't remember at all."

"His initials are G.B. Does that help? His first name begins with a G and his last name begins with B."

"No, it doesn't help."

"His first name is George," Corkin said. "What's his last name?"

"G.B.," H.M. repeated, but otherwise stayed silent, apparently straining to think.

"I'm going to give you three to choose from, and tell me which one it is. Is it George Burns, George Brown, or George Bush?"

"President Bush."

"How do you feel about answering so many questions and doing all the tests that we give you?"

"I don't mind. What is found out about me helps you to help others."

Today, Corkin was trying to address the question of whether a person can be said to have "a sense of self" in the absence of memory. Corkin pointed to H.M.'s "altruism" as evidence of his sense of self. He was endlessly cooperative for the teams of researchers who arrived at MIT to run one test or another on him, taking pleasure in the idea that "what is found out about me helps you to help others." Plus, Corkin said, there were other things about H.M., other values, other characteristics that demonstrated his intact person-ness. For instance, his "realistic goals."

"It turns out he wanted to be a brain surgeon," she said. "He tells you this quite often, then he says, 'but I couldn't, because I wear glasses, and when the nurse wiped my brow she might disrupt my glasses and then I wouldn't see properly and I would go in and damage the brain and hurt the person and I don't want to do that.'"

I reflected on Corkin's true sportsmanship in attempting to fit her research findings, her whole way of thinking, into this particular psychoanalytic forum, using what she imagined to be relevant information to answer the vague question "What defines a self?" It was the kind of question she wouldn't have had to deal with in her lab at MIT, where investigations were confined to the highly specific and easily quantifiable. For instance: How many digits could H.M. hold in his short-term memory? For how long between presentations of stimuli could H.M.'s working memory preserve the information: fifteen seconds, thirty seconds, or sixty seconds? Of course, all such questions are asked in the service of a much larger exploration: an inquiry into the very functions that define us as human. Yet this sense of grandeur is often lost, perhaps necessarily, in the questions themselves.

"One thing that I was thinking about was how would Freud have defined 'self,'" Corkin said at one point in the conference. "And in my simpleminded way, I thought, well, it's probably that you make a composite of id, ego, and superego, and then you get some sort of a weighted average of the information and extract something out that you call 'self.'" An awkward pause followed Corkin's interpretation of psychoanalytic theory.

To the psychoanalysts present in the audience, I knew, Corkin's remarks about H.M. would seem lacking in depth, helpful in a lab but insufficient for conveying a textured sense of the man himself, with his inner life brimming in the subtext. Corkin and the psychoanalysts were looking through two different lenses. Indeed, Corkin acknowledges as much in her 2013 book about the life of H.M., *Permanent Present Tense*. Corkin writes that although H.M. began participating in neuropsychological studies in 1962, measuring every aspect of his memory, performance, and behavior, no one thought to test his "emotional state" until the early 1980s. She explains: "We had not done this evaluation previously because in the 1960s and 1970s, many neuroscientists, including members of my lab, shunned topics that belonged in the realm of clinical psychology and psychiatry." Corkin does not expand on this terse statement, yet her scant words say almost everything there is to be said about the dividing lines running between the study of the brain and the mind. Even though Corkin's colleagues were determined to understand H.M.'s brain, for at least twenty years they were not inclined to believe that understanding his "mind" could be relevant.

And here, now, in Montreal, 2008, the culture clash continued. Almost as soon as Corkin had mentioned H.M.'s wistful dream of becoming a brain surgeon, there were signs that the audience was growing restive. Hands waved for the mic. A French psychoanalyst sprang to her feet.

"His professional ideals, like being a neurosurgeon, I just don't believe it at all," she declared, in her Parisian accent. "This is a fantasy. I think also there is a lot of aggression in himself. I don't think he's so nice, either."

Corkin considered this. "Maybe not deep deep deep deep deep down," she allowed, diplomatically.

The French analyst was about to make a further remark when Corkin continued, "Let me just add something now. And that is, does he show extremes of affect? And the answer is yes, but not very often. So when his father died, his uncle came to take away his prized gun collection, and he got very angry."

"Well," the French analyst said, "he would like to shoot the neurosurgeon."

Corkin looked baffled. The analyst, satisfied, sat down.

Once again, I considered the strange charms of the psychoanalytic profession.

And still, Corkin was game. "The other thing is, he did have recurrent dreams and I know this is very important for you guys," she said. "In 1977, I did nine nights of all-night sleep studies."

I could detect a collective drawing of breath. H.M.'s dreams? This was brand new.

"I don't feel very secure with these data, because there was no way to validate whether it was a dream or whether he was just trying to be a cooperative subject and make up a nice story for this examiner," Corkin said.

She explained that for the nine nights they studied H.M.'s sleep and dreams, she had two different graduate students, alternating nights, wake H.M. up when the EEG recording indicated REM sleep—when dreaming most often occurs—and ask whether or not he had been dreaming. Corkin was concerned when she noticed that one of the graduate students, the one with whom H.M. had far more personal rapport, was able to elicit more detail from H.M. about his dream life than the other. This, Corkin felt, showed a fatal flaw in the methodology. Science cannot depend on personal rapport. So she took her nine nights' worth of data and locked them in a drawer.

It wasn't long before Mark Solms reached for the microphone. He looked rather eager, like a kid in a classroom, bursting to be called upon.

"I want to say how very fortunate we've been to have Dr. Corkin here," he said. "She's the main guardian and investigator of probably the most famous case in the history of neuropsychology, and to come from completely outside of our field and so generously share your unique experience with us, we're very, very grateful." Solms paused, then turned the full force of his boyish charm upon Corkin. "And while you're feeling warmly disposed towards us, I want to quickly tell you that I am the man to study the dream material."

Around me, I noticed people smiling indulgently. Soon, I would understand just exactly what Solms had meant.

4

The reproaches against science for not having yet solved the problems of the universe are exaggerated in an unjust and malicious manner; it has truly not had time enough yet for these great achievements. Science is very young—a human activity which developed late.

—SIGMUND FREUD, 1933

FALL 2008

Three months later, I was on my way to Washington, D.C., having fled the red barn in New Hampshire, to which I'd recently moved. I was now beginning to work as a freelance journalist; I was on assignment to cover the annual conference of the Society for Neuroscience. It was being held in the D.C. convention center, a place as vast and impersonal as an airport. Ten days before, Obama had been elected president. Now, just a mile from the White House, I was entering into a completely different reality. Around me, the cavernous halls were mobbed with neuroscientists rushing to presentations to absorb their colleagues' latest findings or to represent their own. I was already late—late to the Rockefeller Institute's rollout of their findings on stress and the brain. I was wondering where I could get some gum. The morning had unveiled the news that with a stick of Juicy Fruit, I could hope to boost my short-term memory and become 240 percent less stressed in the process. Never mind that the Wrigley Science Institute had funded the study. It was just one of thousands of papers that had lured more than thirty thousand people to Washington.

Despite the activity, the convention center was strangely quiet, the tall windows admitting a dreary gray light. The attendees were mostly young, many of them grad students and postdocs. Ostensibly, this was a fantastic singles scene, but I didn't pick up on much sexual ambition beneath the exchanges. It didn't matter. I had a story to file and a list of sessions that the SfN press office had specifically suggested that I, and the other journalists here, attend, sessions expected to lend themselves to media-friendly consumption, sessions devoted to, for instance: "Sexual Identity in Mice," "The Neurobiology of Decision Making," and the "Neurological Basis of Love." Each day was packed with presentations on every imaginable subject in current neuroscientific research. The complete program consumed five floppy volumes, which I carted around in a canvas tote bag until my shoulders gave out. The lectures were held in rooms so large I couldn't see the speaker. Instead, I watched heads projected onto giant screens. I perused the details of study designs, followed the path of red-light laser pointers dancing around tables of p-values, as if a world of innovation lurked just inside. Perhaps it did. The schedule was strict. No time to loiter. No time to engage.

I was covering this conference for a news publication where I'd recently begun to work. It was my idea to come: this meeting was the single occasion of the year on which it seemed possible to achieve something like an unobstructed view of the ever-expanding field. Far-flung scientists gathered to discuss what now, what next.

I imagined that being here was like visiting Palo Alto in 1993, or whenever it was that the future changed.

Around me, hundreds of attendees massed in exhausted clumps along the carpeted hallways, sitting cross-legged, staring into laptop screens, and wolfing down cheeseburgers to fortify themselves for the next presentation, the next session, the next meeting. As each day wore on, my surroundings began to feel more and more like a Las Vegas casino, a self-contained universe where time did not exist and oxygen was pumped in to dissuade you from leaving.

In the swarm of information, I didn't know what to suggest to my editor. I was reporting on a shifting landscape. Everything was novel, everything a potential breakthrough. Yet who was to say how it would turn out? What would and what wouldn't ultimately matter? And should those criteria even be relevant when thinking about what was interesting right now?

The real action, I discovered, the unscripted buzz, was unfolding downstairs in the basement. Here, the poster sessions took place, laying out the fine grain details of neuroscientific advance. In front of each poster stood a scientist prepared to explain himself to anyone interested in asking. I stopped to squint at "Cocaine and the Firing Patterns of the Nucleus Accumbens" (a brain structure linked to reward and addiction), but only for a minute or two, before continuing through the endless maze that shifted twice a day, every day, as the a.m. posters were taken down and replaced by the p.m. batch. There were more than twenty thousand posters on display that week.

What I was seeing play out around me was the self-correcting clause that is written into science. Even the most senior, most seasoned neuroscientists could be spotted roaming these aisles, stopping to fix their laser gaze on the methodological assumptions of a young PhD candidate from some obscure lab they'd never heard of. It was a democracy of purpose. The energy was palpable. Here, for me, was the true ground zero of those actually at work on the future.

A Danish researcher stood before her poster on "White Matter Lesions in Depression." With fMRI images, she illustrated her conclusion that depression was associated with lesions in the brain—but, she conceded, her findings were still inconclusive. She told me that her work was driven by the goal to establish depression as a physical illness, with physical symptoms and causes. If this could be accomplished, she believed, depression would gain legitimacy as a neurobiological disease. Her poster typified a truism of neuroscientific research: in the search for answers, the questions had to be shrunk down to their smallest components.

And here again, I entertained a familiar refrain: *What about the rest?* It was a thought I wouldn't have articulated aloud, since I saw that the spirit of the inquiry ran contrary to the scientific process, grinding forward at its steady pace of piece by piece. Yet I was always bumping up against what felt like the limits of what any one psychological theory or scientific hypothesis or neurochemical schema could hope to explain about a person. This was glaringly true, for instance, in the case of my father, who had, over the last several months, surprised us all by emerging from his three-year-long internal disappearance, regaining animation for reasons that he himself couldn't necessarily grasp. "Music," he would later say, "and books. And my own determination." And pills, and doctors, and sitting on a leather sofa on East Fifty-Eighth Street, talking to a psychologist with an amazing name: Stratyner. And time itself. Somewhere, in this swirling concoction, a path to recovery had materialized. But recovery from what, I now had occasion to wonder. For the very concept of disease implied some clear dividing line between who my father was before, during, and after the years in question. Well, I'd never seen such a line.

"I haven't learnt to dissect a prairie vole that way, but I intend to," remarked a young woman as I continued down the aisle. "It's a weak point in my research. I know that." She had on thick mascara and tall boots. Hers was one of many posters, I was noticing, that featured prairie voles. This was because prairie voles are one of the few naturally monogamous animal species. For their fidelity, they had become a hot animal model, widely sought out by scientists studying such phenomena as the brain chemistry of intimacy and attachment.

Near the prairie voles, a Japanese researcher stood before his discovery: pre-germinated brown rice is good for the brain. I saw another group of Japanese researchers unveiling "Mirror and Makeup in Facial Perception." According to their poster, they had investigated the question of "the self as seen by the self" and "the self as seen by others." There was a gap between the two, they were arguing. They concluded that using makeup bridges this gap. The researcher's nametag spelled out his corporate affiliation: Kanebo Cosmetics, Inc. I was surprised that such blatant commercial interests were represented here, lurking among the scientific posters, and as I continued to wind my way through the aisles, I found that it had become more difficult to know what was legitimate science, what was corporate advertising, and what exactly constituted the gray zone in between. To my eyes, the information on offer was presented in an undifferentiated flood.

Another day, another poster session, another Japanese researcher— this one presenting his findings on the effect of antidepressants on the brain. He had found that antidepressants boost the levels of BDNF, an important growth protein. Directly next to his poster, a second poster reported exactly the opposite conclusion. Antidepressants have no effect on BDNF, it stated. I pointed this out to him. He smiled demurely. We looked for the other researcher, but she was not in the vicinity. When I came back an hour later, I found the two of them engaged in an amiable conversation, each explaining away their own data to accommodate the other's position. I stepped in, with the intention of galvanizing some sort of confrontation, but they would not be provoked. Consensus had formed here. I moved on.

On the final day, the crowd thinning, I migrated with the droves to Union Station. Many of them were still wearing nametags, their poster tubes strapped to their backs like yoga mats. It was time for them to redeploy to their labs in Philadelphia, New York, Boston, and beyond, to take up their positions at microscopes and scanning machines. There were flags to be planted, a cosmic riddle to be solved. Sitting on the northbound Amtrak train, I reflected for perhaps the hundredth time that week that it was difficult to see how someone like Mark Solms fit into the neuroscientific landscape. To say "Freud" to scientists engaged in the pursuit of empirical truths was to risk making yourself instantly suspect and quickly irrelevant.

Yet I was troubled by how many people appeared to be participating in the reducing down of the brain's most complicated questions with little apparent regard for the long history of clinical insight established by psychoanalysis and psychiatry. The rush of findings about the brain that was permeating our current moment seemed to me like a new reality we would define ourselves by, and then wouldn't be able to turn back from. And I didn't want to subscribe to a version of life where creativity is explained as patterns of electrical waves, sadness as the number you circle between one and nine, and love confused with the mating habits of prairie voles. I had, I discovered, become attached to an unfashionable cause with uncertain prospects. I had just spent four days staring into the formidably unbothered heart of modern neuroscience. I didn't know what the chances could be for someone who was bent on insisting that these same scientists take seriously the question of our inner lives.

5

SPRING 2009

It was the middle of the night when we landed in Dakar. I was wired, wide awake among the sleeping bodies, stuffed into what must have been an especially tiny middle seat, staring at the screen in front of me as it tracked our descent into Senegal. As the plane sat on the tarmac waiting to refuel, I walked to the back in my socks, stuck my head out the open door into the inky black night: first breath drawn in Africa. I was ecstatic and terrified. I was twenty-six. I was en route to Cape Town to spend time with Mark Solms. I believed that I had to understand the full scope of this person in order to understand his work. "The personal and the scientific are always, hopefully, fused," writes Oliver Sacks. And this sentiment, this credo, was the great theme of Solms's own work: the inextricability of the person from the pathology, the psyche from the neurons, the mind from the brain. Since meeting Solms the year before, I'd come to think that the work he was doing told a revealing story about neuroscience. It was a story I'd become preoccupied with trying to tell. I was determined to speak to the sense I had that something important, something crucial, was being left out of the study of the brain, and I wanted Solms to be my protagonist. And so I was on my way to Cape Town, even though it was not at all clear whether I was fully expected or, for that matter, exactly welcome there.

"You're coming to Cape Town next weekend?" Solms had said to me, incredulously, when I'd seen him in New York the week before.

"Well, yes."

"Well, we can't just leave it like that!"

Well, we didn't. On my second day in Cape Town, I was up early, driving to Groote Schuur Hospital, following the careful directions that Solms had called to give me. The hospital sloped up a steep hill in the middle of the city. Turning in from the main road, I passed a cemetery, then, just above it, the emergency room, before climbing to the main campus at the top. I walked through the airy courtyard set down amid elegant English colonial buildings. It all felt vaguely tropical, because of the palm trees.

I was early, but Solms was earlier, smoking a cigarillo at a picnic table outside the neurological unit. Across from him sat his assistant, Eleni, warm, youthful, dressed in a fur-lined vest and stilettos. On the table between them, a cardboard box was brimming with loose sheets of paper. Eleni carted this box everywhere, I would soon discover. It was a perpetual presence. It was Solms's portable inbox. It was their Sisyphean pursuit. They were chipping away at it when I arrived.

"You can't miss the faculty meeting. Really, Mark, you can't, you missed the last one," Eleni was just in the midst of saying. Solms, looking beleaguered, stuffed out his cigarillo for emphasis. Then we headed inside, through a lackadaisical metal detector that seemed not to be plugged in, down a hallway, down another. Solms walked quickly and Eleni kept pace. Groote Schuur was a teaching hospital, linked to the University of Cape Town, where Solms was chair of the neuropsychology department. It was here at Groote Schuur, decades before, that the surgeon Christiaan Barnard performed the world's first successful human heart transplant; it was also to here that Solms's brother, Lee, was flown, at age six, when he fell off a roof and crushed his skull. Now this was where Mark Solms saw his own brain-injured patients.

Inside the hospital I noticed certain details: there was no soap in the bathrooms, and no soap canisters, either, no plans for soap. Solms waved to the nurses—"the sisters"—and punched a code to unlock the door to his office. Four different video cameras were bolted down on various surfaces, aimed at the desk, to capture from every angle whatever took place there.

Solms's graduate students swarmed in cheerfully, all in their twenties. They would be qualified as neuropsychologists in a year or two.

"Watch closely," Solms said, flipping open the file of the patient we would soon be shadowing him to see. "Her name is Arena Thomas, and she's Afrikaans-speaking, but we will hope she can speak English, if only for the sake of our visitor, who speaks no Afrikaans.

"Day before yesterday, she woke up with a left-sided hemiparesis, with slurred speech, with confusion, and with reduced level of consciousness," Solms continued. "So all we're going to do is go and look at her, and what we will expect to find is an acute right-hemisphere stroke who will behave like an acute right-hemisphere stroke, and we all know what to expect: the patient is nothing like what you expect."

We hurried to keep up with Solms as he blazed down the hall and into the inner chambers of the neurological ward. We passed through a succession of open rooms, rows of patients lying in beds, or sitting semi-erect in chairs next to their beds. The floor was suffused with an eerie absence of noise. It felt like uninhabited space. To look at any of the patients was to see someone in another dimension who was no longer a part of reality as you experienced it. I felt the usual compulsion to avert my eyes, out of courtesy, or fear. When I did look into a patient's face, I imagined I saw an accusation, which I later understood as my own guilt, because I was able to go gliding by, while they were stuck there, having lost everything.

Solms held a curtain open for us to pass through in a single file, forming a tight ring around the bed of the patient, Mrs. Thomas. We were pressed in almost to the point of touching her mattress. There was nothing to do but look right at her. Mrs. Thomas, propped up on her pillows, had jutting cheekbones, missing teeth, and weary, wrinkled eyes. She looked us all over once, and then shifted her attention permanently back to Solms, who was standing by her head. He leaned his torso down at an angle approaching ninety degrees, putting his face just above hers, and, greeting her warmly in Afrikaans, asked if she spoke English.

"Yes. It's a diverse country," she said in English, with slurry satisfaction.

She was lucid, if drowsy. She was also, it seemed, strangely amused.

Solms beamed back at her.

"Do you know why you're here? Do you know how you got here?" he asked.

Mrs. Thomas did and did not know. Her nose wouldn't stop bleeding, she remembered. She didn't know that she had had a major stroke; she was not clear about why she still needed to be in the hospital. She made no mention at all of the fact that she couldn't move the left side of her body.

"We're going to do everything we can to make you better, you are in the best hospital in the country," Solms assured her. He was stroking her arms and hands as he spoke with her, as if to anchor her attention to herself. He began to ask her questions, poking about to get a sense of where things stood with her. Gradually, bits and pieces of her story emerged, the wispy images of someone's life. Her children were dead. She lived with her ex-husband; she did not work. She was more than anything else preoccupied with the question of her dog. Who would care for her dog while she was in the hospital?

"What's your dog's name?" Solms asked.

"Blondie," she said, and the dog came into focus.

Solms bantered with her about the dog and she followed along, happily cooperative. He stroked her right hand. "Can you move your right hand, Mrs. Thomas?" he asked. She lifted her right hand. "Now your left hand," he said. "Can you move your left hand for me?"

We were staring at her left arm, lying immobile on top of the blanket. The hand was balled up in a fist. She didn't move it. She didn't look at it. She didn't say, "Oh my god, what's wrong with my arm?" Instead, she maintained her air of vague bemusement and kept her gaze trained on Solms.

"I love my left hand," she finally remarked. "My mother was ambidextrous."

"Have you inherited that from her?" Solms asked.

"I hope not," she answered.

"Why?"

"It was unnerving. She had one hand on the butter and one hand on the jam."

Solms tried to return her attention to her left hand, but Mrs.

Thomas was unwilling to discuss it. She was becoming rapidly fatigued, withdrawing bit by bit into a sleepy remove. To every question Solms asked about her left arm, she replied noncommittally. Yes, everything was fine with her left arm, why shouldn't it be? Or she would simply ignore the question and lapse into a dreamy silence. This went on for minutes, Solms repeatedly inquiring about her left arm. He tried one final time, stroking her left hand vigorously with his own. There was silence as she finally looked down at it. It was an awkward silence, the kind that surrounds the inevitable moment when the pleasantries have been exchanged and you're forced to state your business. Mrs. Thomas's arm did not move. We stared at it. Still, it did not move.

"Don't be cross, doctor," Mrs. Thomas said. "I'll do it for you later."

She had curled up as though to sleep.

"Do you have any other questions for me?" Solms asked her.

"What's your name?"

"Mark Solms."

"You've left your mark!" she told him, grinning, flashing her missing teeth good-naturedly.

Back in Solms's office, we regained our seats.

"Okay, what's her most striking symptom?" Solms asked.

"Anosognosia," the students said in a chorus.

"That's the first anosognosia you've seen, isn't it?" Solms said. "So it's your unsullied, untainted, virginal impression."

Anosognosia—or, "lack of awareness of one's illness"—is not very subtle, it turns out.

A student asked Solms why he had seemed to be so adamantly

pushing back against Mrs. Thomas's inability or refusal to acknowledge what was happening to her body; why he had asked so many times for her to try to move her left hand, or to admit that she couldn't.

"You don't just go along with the denial," Solms said. "I'm speaking to the underlying awareness that there's something the matter."

Solms was choosing his words carefully. He was speaking from a psychoanalytic viewpoint, but he didn't use the vocabulary. He said "underlying awareness" instead of "unconscious." He dodged a language that came with certain implications.

"Her comment 'I love my left hand'—that's absolutely characteristic," he said. "They have very strange attitudes to their left hands; we could have gotten more out of that. If you sit with her for an hour, my prediction is you'll find all sorts of strange ideas about her hand and its connection to the dog and to the cat and to her son. If a psychoanalyst sat there and explored those things, that's the direction you're heading in."

Here in this room at Groote Schuur Hospital, Solms was a professor of neuropsychology. Everyone seemed to know, vaguely, that Professor Solms was a psychoanalyst, somewhere else, in a different part of his life, but that fact didn't quite connect up to the immediate reality of the neurological ward. No one asked him to elaborate on what else a psychoanalyst might explore should a psychoanalyst be present at Mrs. Thomas's bedside.

Indeed, Solms's life was, I was beginning to see, divided into compartments. It had been with a sense of surprise a few months before that I had discovered on Google that Solms owned and lived on a fully functioning vineyard in Franschhoek, an hour outside the city. He had bought Solms-Delta in 2001, when he'd moved his family from London back to South Africa. His house was in the

Cape Dutch style, bright white with the characteristic curls, laid out around a square courtyard. I recognized it right away from the photographs I'd seen online. When I came up the dusty driveway for the first time in the distorting glare of the afternoon sun, rows and rows of trussed-up plants, future grapes, seemed to roll out directly from the back door of the house towards the thick forest in the distance. The beauty of the land overwhelmed me.

Solms came back, he often says, because of the "ethical weight" of being South African, of feeling that, after apartheid, it was his moral responsibility to return to the country where he had been educated—where he had reaped all the benefits of being white in a country rigged in his favor—and participate in its future. Now, he runs the Solms-Delta vineyard on a model of parity: when he arrived, he restructured the farm as a cooperative, with all the workers owning a share. Solms has received a great deal of attention nationally and internationally for the many and various policies he's put into place, trying for something like social justice, if only on his one plot of land.

In an idle moment during my first visit there, I wandered alone as far as good manners would allow, through the adjoining analytic offices kept by Solms and his wife, Karen Kaplan-Solms, also a psychoanalyst. They were gracious, wood-paneled rooms, with the requisite Oriental carpets and analytic couches. Solms's couch was covered, like the floor all around it, with precarious towers of hardcover Freud and piles and piles of manuscript pages. I assumed that these were all connected to the task I knew Solms was immersed in: the complete revision of James Strachey's official translation of the Standard Edition of Freud. Solms had been doing it in his off-hours. He had been at it for more than a decade.

On the wall, a framed letter read:

7 Nov 1993
Dear Doctor Solms,
Thanks for the delightful hour. Analysis is in safe hands with you.

It was signed "KR Eissler," the revered and feared psychoanalyst who had stood guard, Cerberus-like, over the Freud archives for an entire generation.

"For years I would wake up every morning and think, I'm Mark Solms, I'm alive, but I haven't finished the Standard Edition and I don't know how I'm going to, and I can see why everyone else has died on the job," Solms would tell me.

In 1984, Solms, aged twenty-three, read the following footnote in a book by Frank Sulloway called *Freud, Biologist of the Mind:* "The difficulties that have long beset students of Freud will be greatly alleviated by the forthcoming publication, in three volumes, of *The Pre-Analytical Works of Sigmund Freud.*"

Solms, a graduate student in Johannesburg, was schooling himself in Freudian theory. Already a qualified neuropsychologist, he was fascinated by the lesser-known history of Freud's attempts to grapple with neurology, in the years before he turned his full attention to the psychological. "Pre-analytical works" refers to everything Freud had done during his two decades in the hard sciences, leading up to the end of the nineteenth century. There was, Solms knew, a considerable amount of it. The Sulloway biography had been published in 1979. Surely, Solms reasoned, those pre-analytic translations would by now be finished. Solms went to his local bookshop, which was run by an erudite Dutchman, who put in an order to the publisher, Hogarth Press, in London. But the order was never filled.

At first, Solms attributed this to the academic boycotts that were so commonly enacted against South Africa throughout the 1980s. Finally, he wrote to the publisher himself to inquire. John Charlton wrote back to inform Solms that the translator had died and the project had been left incomplete. Solms wrote again. Could he see whatever material had been finished? This was how Solms went from being someone who wanted to buy the translations, to being someone who was charged with producing them, as he likes to say.

By 1988, Solms and his wife were living in London, Solms training at the Institute of Psychoanalysis and working on his translations of Freud's neuroscientific papers on the side. He went back and forth to Vienna, digging through the archives for medical journals from the nineteenth century, hunting down any articles Freud might have published there. Solms was slipping into the world of Freud scholarship.

"Their whole lives are sitting like gnomes in libraries and finding these obscure three lines that Freud contributed," Solms said, describing his various counterparts. But he, too, was impassioned about what he was doing. He began to hear murmurs among the Freud crowd that there were problems with James Strachey's translations. Until now, the Strachey translations were the single comprehensive version of Freud in English that Freud himself had approved, reviewing with Strachey various semantic choices carefully before Strachey began his work. Strachey had published the Standard Edition in bursts, working all through the 1950s and into the '60s, after Freud's death, when Strachey himself was entering old age.

"He literally went blind in the process," Solms said.

Freud wrote by hand, in penmanship that could be almost illegible. Strachey had overlooked sentences, left out paragraphs. Moreover, there was controversy among psychoanalysts and other people who cared, avidly, about these things, regarding certain choices Strachey had made. For instance, the issue of *der Trieb*. Freud uses the German word *Trieb* all throughout his forty years of analytic texts, naturally, because it means "drive," a concept to which Freud devoted much attention. But when Strachey sat down to do his English translations, he translated *Trieb* as "instinct." This, Solms knew, was a significant distortion of Freud's intended meaning, because instinct and drive are not interchangeable concepts. Instincts have objects, by definition. They are the biologically inherited reactions we have to specific objects in our environment. For instance, a cat's instinct to pounce on a mouse. A mouse's instinct to flee from a cat. A drive, by contrast, is an urge without an object, an impulse to seek, a libidinal attraction towards something inchoate and unspecified, towards "I know not what," as Solms says. The drive exists on its own terms, even before it has an aim.

There was a general consensus that Strachey's Standard Edition needed updating. And, Solms heard, an Englishman named Albert Dickson had been at work on the project for more than a decade. Solms asked the publisher, John Charlton, whether he could take a look at Dickson's progress. He was surprised to discover that Dickson didn't seem to have any knowledge of psychoanalytic theory. He had had no analytic training and, as it turned out, he appeared not to know the import of the language he was busy rearranging. He didn't understand the implications of the word choices *superego* versus *over-ego* versus *over-I*. He didn't know that analysts had been squinting at this diction for decades, searching with an exacting eye for clues about how to run their clinical practices, like judicial clerks searching for legal precedents. Dickson couldn't detect the full weight that came attached to every word Freud wrote.

And then one night, Dickson's flat burned down, with Dickson inside of it. Solms, now in his early thirties, inherited the job.

"You know, there are many things like that in life," Solms told me. "You would never take them on if you knew what you were really in for."

6

I am only now beginning to grasp how the past persists in
the present, how the present incorporates the past.

—MARK SOLMS, NOTEBOOKS, 1992

SOLMS HAS A MAGNETIC PULL. People uproot their lives and come
to South Africa to enter into his orbit. While I was there, there were
two examples of this, both named George—Georg Schönbächler, a
Swiss scientist and expert on neuropeptides, and Gyuri Fodor, from
Vienna, a psychoanalyst who had moved to Cape Town four years
earlier with his wife and three children. He came when he discovered Solms's work and wrote to Solms and arranged to meet him,
"to make sure he wasn't a fraud," as Fodor put it to me, with the
outsized pride of a certain kind of art collector.

Fodor had wavy brown hair, hooded eyes, and the bone structure of a hawk. He dressed with instinctive insouciance, European
chic. I had met him the year before at the Montreal conference; he
had become part of Solms's initiative to foster neuropsychoanalysis
around the world. When I was in Cape Town, Fodor was preparing
to begin a study that Solms had designed: psychoanalyzing a population of patients with Urbach-Wiethe disease, an extremely rare
genetic disorder in which a person's amygdala gradually calcifies
until it is almost completely defunct. There happened to be a rela-

tively large community of them living together in a poor, depressed region about four hours away from Cape Town. For Solms, these people afflicted with a rare disorder represented exactly the kind of opportunity he was constantly trying to persuade his psychoanalyst colleagues to seize: brains with clearly demarcated failings. The assumption—thus far untested by Solms and his colleagues—was that without their brain's "threat detector," people would lose all fear and inhibition, no longer able to perceive danger. Solms was particularly interested in what effect this might have on the content of their dreams. He wanted to know what could be learned in psychoanalytic terms about what happens when someone's amygdala turns to stone.

One morning during my time in South Africa, I was in the backseat of Mark Solms's silver Volvo, driving with him from Groote Schuur to the University of Cape Town. Up front sat Georg Schönbächler, the Swiss neuropeptide expert, who was taking that year in Cape Town to work with Solms. It was only a short drive, but we were stuck in terrible traffic, Third World traffic, swaddled in exhaust fumes. The sun was pouring into our hot car. I could feel Solms's frustration mounting.

"Come on, be a bus!" he shouted at the bus stalled out in front of us.

Suddenly, Solms turned his laser beam on me. His green eyes narrowed into inquisitive slits in his rearview mirror. "But what exactly is your book about?" he asked. "How will I make sure that the verboten stays verboten?"

Since early that morning when I'd first appeared at Groote Schuur, Solms had been acting wary and peevish, as if he were only now aware of me hovering on the periphery with my spiral notebook and my tape recorder. I wasn't sure what I'd done, specifically, to make him apprehensive, but I tended towards reticence when anyone asked me anything about what exactly I was doing. Afraid to expose my uncertainty, I hid behind a mask of journalistic remove. Solms had finally gotten agitated with me.

"What do you think?" Solms said, turning toward Georg—that moment's coconspirator—after I'd spluttered out a few vague explanations from the backseat. "Should we fire her?"

I felt myself turning red. Solms's eyes mocked me in the rearview mirror. "Look, look, how panicky she's getting," he said to Georg. "She sees her whole book evaporating."

I dropped my hasty attempt to explain myself. I didn't have a simple answer. But why should I? To hell with him then, I thought, as I stared out the window in a disassociated state.

"Don't worry, don't worry," Solms said after a few more moments of silence. "I'm only half kidding. I'm not nearly the narcissist you think I am."

Solms grew up in a world the size of a raindrop. He was born in Namibia, in a tiny town called Lüderitz on the edge of the country, right next to the ocean. Namibia, which sits just above South Africa on the Western edge of the continent, was a German colony for much of the nineteenth century, and German was still widely spoken there when Solms was growing up.

Namibia is desert. It is the second-least densely populated country on earth. In the first years of the twentieth century, the discovery of diamonds on the country's Skeleton Coast transformed the landscape into the object of maniacal extraction. German émigrés rushed in, self-appointed heirs to Africa's riches. Lüderitz, perfectly placed, swelled with new, white inhabitants. The Skeleton Coast became known as the *Sperrgebiet,* which is German for "forbidden territory."

"They roped it off. It was a country within a country," Solms said. "And a company called De Beers took charge of it."

It was a typical Solms remark. "A company called De Beers": ironic, punchy, slightly diminishing. De Beers, of course, is the world's major diamond purveyor, the supplier to countless royals and celebrities, responsible for so many of the engagement rings twinkling all over Manhattan.

But by the time Solms was born, the Skeleton Coast diamonds had nearly run out, and Lüderitz was a ghostly relic of an earlier era. All the trappings of its former German splendor remained. At the edge of town, abandoned baronial mansions stood empty, entombed in piles of sand blown in from the desert. Solms would scale the sand dunes and crawl inside the buried houses, down their grand, decaying staircases into the padded darkness below.

It was easy for me to see in Solms vestiges of the boy who looked out from the empty mansions to which he'd laid claim, onto the infinite yellow-red blankness of the Namib desert, and believe the world to be his, all his. Certainly the political situation at the time reinforced this assumption. Solms's father, Douglas, was the administrator of the Skeleton Coast's remaining diamond supply. He was an employee of the Consolidated Diamond Mines corporation, or CDM, which owned all of the *Sperrgebiet* diamonds, as well as most of the diamonds in South Africa. CDM, which was owned by the Oppenheimer family, represents itself in glass cases as De Beers. Everyone who lived in Lüderitz was a CDM employee, or related to a CDM employee. The region was virtually closed to outsiders, who required special permission to visit. Tourists were prohibited.

A regular feature of life in Lüderitz was the trip, in a five-seater plane, over swaths of empty desert, to a town called Oranjemund in the southwestern corner of Namibia, just above what is today the South African border. Oranjemund was Lüderitz's sibling outpost; there was a school there, and doctors, and a yacht club where Solms's parents went sailing.

When Mark's older brother, Lee, had his accident, tumbling headfirst off the roof of the Oranjemund yacht club, Sylvia Solms, their mother, was appalled by the report that ran in the newspaper. The article stated that Sylvia had left the children alone in order "to rehearse." In truth, Solms tells me, his parents weren't on dry land when Lee crashed into concrete. They were sailing.

"They were hedonists!" Solms often says at this point in the story, and this is a story that Solms often tells. Yet every time I heard it, it somehow seemed less clear. There was, first of all, the question of how a four- and six-year-old came to be alone on a roof. Or at least Solms is nearly certain he was on that roof. He has just the slightest hint of a memory of seeing his brother fall. What would he have seen had he crawled to the edge and looked down to where Lee now lay, unmoving, on the concrete surface below, having suffered a massive cerebral hemorrhage that would change all of their lives?

Afterwards, there was a family code of silence on the subject of what had happened to Lee. When he came back, in a helicopter, from a month of surgery at Groote Schuur, no one in the family acknowledged that Lee had damaged his brain. Sylvia Solms would say: "He's just like me—he's not an intellectual." Mark's own, normal development was in a certain subtle way discouraged. *You mustn't outdo your brother.*

The details of this life don't flow from Solms as the stories from his later years do. Solms is a natural storyteller, fluent and animated. But when the conversation turns to this period, he enters into an uncharacteristic fog. When I asked him one day how far Oranjemund is from Lüderitz, he looked puzzled.

"Eight miles?" he finally said.

"But you flew there in a plane."

"Hm, yes, that's right! So it couldn't have been eight miles."

The actual distance is one hundred and fifty miles. Solms would have made that trip, Lüderitz to Oranjemund, more than a hundred times before he turned fourteen and left for boarding school.

At his school for boys in Pretoria, Solms read in the newspaper of the events in Soweto. It was June 1976. A group of students in the country's largest township, just outside of Johannesburg, had refused to go to school. They were protesting, most specifically, a new decree that their education be taught in Afrikaans, the language of the apartheid regime. The atmosphere in Soweto was so combustible that the students' gesture spread across the township within hours. By afternoon, hundreds were marching, most of them school-aged, through the streets, singing protest songs. By the end of the day, the South African police had arrived on the scene, opened fire, and killed scores of people. The riots would last, on and off, for two years, with more than five hundred dead by the end. Solms, at boarding school, had only the dimmest sense of what lay beyond his insulated world. Like the rest of the students, Solms was expected to join the cadets and march around in a brown uniform, the precursor to the mandatory draft that applied to every white male South African. Solms refused. He was called into the headmaster's office. "What's the basis of your objection, Solms?" he was asked. He knew only that he wouldn't, couldn't, participate. "I remember saying it in a half-confused way, not quite knowing whether I really believed this or whether I was just being naughty, or what this was all about," Solms would tell me. For Solms, as for every South African, it would soon be impossible not to know.

.   .   .

It was in this context that Solms arrived at University of the Wit-
watersrand in Johannesburg in 1979. He registered for psychology.
But "psychology was ridiculous," he quickly felt. Psychology as it
was being taught at Wits in the 1980s was essentially behaviorism,
from Skinner on down, theories about reward and punishment,
dogs and bells, rats in mazes. Solms had gone in thinking he was
going to "learn about people," the whole, messy reality of what
it means to have a mind. Instead, he found that psychology was
devoted to breaking the mind down into little parts that bore scant
resemblance to human experience as he knew it. "It was boxes and
arrows!" Solms says, ruefully, semi-disbelievingly, even now.

Disenchanted, Solms switched into neuropsychology. Here still,
he found the same problem: not only was he moored in a reduction-
ist attitude towards the mind, but also, he now found, it was unacceptable to question it. The aspects of human behavior in which
Solms was truly interested were swept under the neuropsychological
rug.

"I had a professor who I asked about these sorts of things. He
basically said, in a nice way, don't ask questions about that. These
are not respectable questions."

A friend told Solms about a seminar in the comparative literature
department on Freud. Solms showed up a few weeks after the start
of the semester, just as the class was assigned Freud's "Project for a
Scientific Psychology." That weekend Solms was house-sitting for
friends, a married couple, who lived off-campus in a house with a
garden. He arrived on Friday with his copy of the Standard Edition of Freud, Volume I. Freud wrote the "Project" in 1896, but it
promptly disappeared, and stayed that way, for the next five decades.

.   .   .

At the time he wrote the "Project," Freud's medical practice was thriving. All through the 1890s, Solms would learn, a steady procession of Viennese hysterics trundled into Freud's consulting room. No one knew what to do with them. Their symptoms included partial paralyses, sudden, uncontrollable twitches, the inexplicable loss of appetite, or being suddenly overwhelmed by a strong scent, which would come out of nowhere and abruptly disappear again. These symptoms were, in a sense, pseudo-neurological: they seemed like the results of the nervous system gone wrong, yet could not be connected to a physical cause—and, indeed, could not be physical: they defied the natural laws of the human body. Freud was riveted. This was weird, and weird was good, because it was a portal to the new, and Freud, above anything else, was wildly ambitious.

By the mid 1890s, he was dealing with the baffling phenomenon of hysteria, but he was thinking, still, like a biologist, rooted in the physical. He had worked in the hard sciences for the last twenty years of his life, publishing papers on such topics as the neuroanatomy of a primitive fish, the gonads of eels (which had been notoriously elusive, but which Freud finally located during a triumphant stint in Trieste), the medicinal properties of cocaine, brain anatomy in humans, and childhood paralyses.

Facing his hysterics, Freud was trying to understand how a brain would have to be built in order to produce the anomalous behaviors he was seeing. And so began the "Project." Freud became obsessed with the effort, sitting down at his desk every night, fueled by cocaine, to struggle with questions that disappeared, eel-like, the moment he thought he'd grasped them. He dispatched letters at a furious rate to his friend in Berlin, Wilhelm Fliess. He thought he had it, he thought he lost it. His attention glistened, his attention drifted.

"Dear Wilhelm," Freud wrote in the fall of 1895, "What a crazy correspondent I am! For two whole weeks I was in a fever of writing and thought I had found the secret, but now I know I have not got it yet, and I have laid the thing aside again."

Finally, after traveling to Berlin to be buoyed up by Fliess, Freud got on the train to go back to Vienna and scribbled most of what is now "Project for a Scientific Psychology" into two empty notebooks. Freud conceived of the work as "a psychology for neurologists." He was trying to create a model of mental function that could incorporate, in one single document, both the brain and the mind. He imagined various categories of "neurones," which worked according to one general principle: avoiding and reducing all forms of excitement. But he quickly grew frustrated with the limits of certainty available to him.

At the time Freud was writing, neurology was in its earliest stages. Even the idea of the neuron itself was controversial at best. This most basic unit of the brain had been discovered only a decade before, by the great Spanish neurologist Santiago Ramón y Cajal. Until Cajal showed, in silvery-stained outline, the tiny, independent cells, many believed that the brain was one continuous, netlike structure. In 1895, there were those still making the case against the neuron, arguing that the brain, which produces such a unified experience of life, couldn't possibly be made up of a billion individual cells, each separate from the other.

When Freud got back to Vienna, he sent his notebooks hurtling through the mail to Fliess, and shortly after decided he never wanted to see them again. He didn't finish "Project for a Scientific Psychology," nor did he publish it. In the end, Freud believed that the "Project" amounted to nothing more than speculation—"imaginings, transpositions, and guesses," as he put it. "Every endeavor to think of ideas as stored up in nerve-cells and of excitations as traveling along nerve-fibers has miscarried completely," he would write. There simply did not yet exist the means to prove one way or the other the theories about the brain that he was putting forward. Neurology was too primitive for Freud's ambitions. He wasn't content to dwell in the limbo of maybe, maybe not, so he dropped the "Project" and the intellectual aims it had represented, and redirected his gaze from the brain to the mind. "We shall remain on psychological ground," Freud declared in *The Interpretation of Dreams,* in 1899. In other words, no more "neurones." But he always said—as Solms often emphasizes—that one day, one day, the neurosciences would be sophisticated enough to take up the observations laid out by psychoanalysis and augment them, prune them, extend them, render them complete.

It wasn't until James Strachey was working on the English Standard Edition of Freud in the 1950s that those two notebooks resurfaced, in Wilhelm Fliess's estate. Strachey promptly translated them and inserted "Project for a Scientific Psychology" into Volume 1 of the Standard Edition, nervously bemoaning, in his introductory remarks, that the original manuscript pages had been unusually illegible (having been written on a moving train).

Solms had encountered nothing like the "Project" before. He went through line by line, cross-referencing it with the seminal neuropsychological text, *The Working Brain* by Alexander Luria, Solms's first great intellectual hero. He positioned both books open on the table in front of him, looking to see how each of Freud's postulations might map onto Luria's later, more definitive model. Solms went back and forth between the two, sentence by sentence,

plumbing the depths of every word. On Sunday night, the door-
bell rang. Solms's friend had come to fetch him. They had dinner
plans. When Solms opened the door, his friend reeled back. "What's
happened?" he asked, staring at Solms, who was overheated and
unshaven and who hadn't exchanged a word with another human
being in three days.

For those who are not ardent followers of the twists and turns
of Freudian thought, the "Project" makes for a difficult read. "The
intention," Freud starts out, "is to furnish a psychology that shall be
a natural science: that is, to represent psychical processes as quan-
titatively determinate states of specifiable material particles, thus
making those processes perspicuous and free from contradiction."
The "Project" is, on the one hand, a deeply technical work, littered
with archaic Greek letters that Freud used to designate his hypo-
thetical categories of neurons. And on the other hand, the "Project"
surprises, following Freud down exotic alleys of new ideas: ideas
about repression, wishes, pain, and pleasure, ideas that thread all the
way through the next forty years of his work.

For Solms, starved as he was for the Bigger Picture, this was
heaven, this was hope. Here was a neuroscientist, just like him,
trained to think of the physical brain itself, looking at it from the
outside in, who was finally grasping at the concepts that had always
seemed to Solms the essence of the matter: the jagged things, the
unlit places.

Solms plunged in, sitting for hours at the university library, reading whatever there was to read by Freud and about Freud. It was
1983. South Africa was politically volatile and intellectually limited.
There was, more or less, no local psychoanalytic tradition to speak
of. There were books, imported from Europe. Solms retreated into
a vacuum of concentration, isolating himself to a large degree from
his current circumstances.

One afternoon, sitting in the library, he looked out the window to see a wave of students crashing by, trailed by the South African police waving their batons and their canisters of tear gas. Solms sat there, watching the riot unfold, and asked himself the obvious question. *What the fuck are you doing?*

There he was, sequestered in an academic sphere of his own making, tracking down archaic developments in nineteenth-century neurology while, all around him, his generation was mobilizing to change the face of their country. But here, in these books, was Solms's future, it was his way up and out, and he knew it. He recognized it even then.

7

Some R hemisphere patients appear to treat their own bodies (or at least their L half) as if they were part of the external world—which in a sense, they are of course. I am grappling with the analogy to melancholia in F (1917). Their rejection of the L side appears to be a component of their more general rejection of the external world (narcissism).

—MARK SOLMS, NOTEBOOKS, 1993

IN SOUTH AFRICA, I was trying to get to the very root of Solms's most important contributions. Twenty-four years old, Solms, newly qualified as a neuropsychologist, went to work in the neurology department at Baragwanath Hospital. Baragwanath, or "Bara," as it's known, is the largest hospital in the world. It sits at the edge of Soweto, connected to the township by a narrow footbridge that arcs over a busy highway. The hospital itself is a sprawling collection of squat brick buildings; the aesthetic, Solms says, is "reminiscent of a concentration camp."

Baragwanath opened in 1942 to provide care for soldiers fighting on behalf of the British in World War II. By the time Solms was working there, Bara was for black patients only, but it retained the atmosphere of wartime conditions, of having to do the best job possible under the circumstances. There was a constant feeling of embattled urgency. There were more than three thousand beds and each one was always taken. At any given time, there were hundreds of patients lying on the floor or slumped in one of the narrow alleys running in between the buildings.

It was 1985 when Solms showed up for his first day of work at Baragwanath. The South African government was teetering on the brink and everybody knew it. White South Africans were leaving the country in droves, particularly those with a professional skill they could rely on to establish new lives somewhere else. Just as Solms was starting out, his supervisor and mentor, Michael Saling, was beginning his new life in Melbourne, Australia, far away from the rioting masses.

Solms found himself in an unusual position. He had just finished his master's degree, he had almost no experience treating patients, and he now constituted the whole of the neuropsychology department at Baragwanath, which served a population of two million people. This was a population that was likelier than most to show up at the emergency room with a grisly brain injury, because life in Soweto was impoverished, miserable, and cramped; people got drunk and brawled; people threw rocks and the police mowed them down with guns. People, thousands of people, came in with screwdrivers sticking out of their heads, shards of glass enmeshed in their skulls, bullets in their brains. A sizeable portion of the doctors on staff were foreign, putting in a stint at Baragwanath for the experience of working with such numerous and extreme cases of traumatic injury. They left experts.

Solms's first day at Baragwanath didn't go so well. The consultant on duty walked Solms through the wards. "I thought, what am I supposed to do? I didn't understand half his words. Am I supposed to memorize all this? I'm going to kill them! I'm going to get it all wrong!" To his eternal horror, Solms collapsed in a dead faint.

In the context of a busy inpatient neurological ward like the one at Baragwanath, the role of the neuropsychologist is more or less limited to diagnosis. A patient comes in—with a stroke, with a bullet wound, with a concussion, with a viral infection, with a severed spinal cord, with a lifetime of alcoholism, with early-onset Alzheimer's, with *something*—and the neuropsychologist administers various tests, and asks various questions, in an attempt to determine what has gone wrong in their brain. If the problem is operable, the patient is sent to surgery; if it's not, the patient goes home.

Solms still remembers his first patient.

"I started assessing him in this awkward way, because I didn't have the proper clinical training," Solms would tell me. "There was something wrong, I could see that, but where's the aphasia and where's the amnesia and where's the apraxia, and how the fuck do you do that? I have no idea.

"I didn't know my ass from my elbow," he recalls, nostalgically.

Solms saw thousands of patients, each one a new strain of catastrophe. It was an immersion education in human fragility. One bump, one bullet, one burst blood vessel, and suddenly our identity is pulled out from beneath us, and we are someone else.

Neuropsychology was still a new field; in South Africa especially, doctors were unfamiliar with the specifics. What was it? It was neuro, but it was also psych; it was a gray zone, where brain merged with mind, what the hell was it? Solms got some strange referrals. People sent him their wayward relatives, probably in some cases hoping for a nice, reasonable, physical explanation for their behavior, something easy to blame.

Often, Solms was clueless, flummoxed by what he was looking at. Every night, he would read up on the day's mysteries, trying to elaborate on the clinical scenarios he had encountered, to begin to understand the way each pattern of damage tended to manifest. It was a haphazard education, Solms left alone to fill in the holes. "You'd see visitors come in, visiting their father or their spouse, and you knew they were written off. That was it. There was no support system for black families in South Africa. Nothing."

Solms was frantically trying to stay afloat, but in truth there wasn't really anyone to hold him accountable for mistakes he might make. There was no superior in the neuropsychology department looking over his shoulder—the person who would have occupied that position was on another continent. More generally, there wasn't a clear understanding in the neurological ward of what exactly it was he was meant to be doing.

At Baragwanath, patients were like a moving ticker tape of neurological tragedy; they appeared, Solms assessed them, and that was typically the last he would see of them. But in the afternoons, Solms returned to white Johannesburg, where he worked in the brain and spine rehabilitation unit of Edenvale General Hospital. Here, people came in the wake of whatever disaster had befallen them and stayed for weeks or months at a time, grappling with their new realities. Solms would see them every day, and get to know them, their full constellation of problems. Their families came to visit, their lives were on display. He was steeped in their worlds, getting a sense, unavoidably, of how their personalities had shifted.

Yet something eluded him.

"There's something about them which is not in the textbooks," he would later say. "I could feel, I knew, they were like *this,* the patients with the right-hemisphere syndromes, they're like *this*—like what? Like *this.* I felt it. But I didn't have a language for it. I didn't have a vocabulary."

The gray zone around neuropsychology served as a cover for

Solms's more experimental tendencies. He announced that he was going to start "doing therapy" with the patients he saw in the rehabilitation clinic. "Nobody thought it was weird, because they didn't *know* it was weird," he would later say. But what did it mean, for Solms, at this stage, to "do therapy"? He had not yet trained as an analyst. But he himself had been in therapy. He knew enough to sit there with the patients and listen to their stories.

The case of Mrs. S.: here was where it started. Johannesburg, 1987. Mrs. S., an Austrian émigré in her sixties, had been in the Edenvale hospital rehabilitation unit since suffering a massive hemorrhage on the right side of her brain a few months before. Now, paralyzed on the left side of her body, she was confined to a wheelchair. But that wasn't why Solms was treating her. She had been referred to him because she was morbidly depressed, and nobody could understand why. Right-hemisphere patients weren't supposed to behave like this. Rather, their traditional presentation was something like what I would observe myself, meeting the patient Mrs. Thomas at Groote Schuur: an implacable, aloof, and uncanny good cheer.

Solms, age twenty-six, walked into the room to discover that his new patient kept at her bedside a framed photograph of herself in full Hitler Youth regalia.

"I've had a right middle cerebral artery thrombotic cerebrovascular accident," she announced to Solms with clipped precision.

Mrs. S., formerly a radiologist, had the exquisitely calibrated vocabulary of a doctor putting the stethoscope on her own condition. Except she made no mention of her left-sided paralysis. Of that, she knew nothing.

Here, for Solms, was a mystery. Why was it that damage to the right side of the brain would result in this peculiar, striking outcome? Mrs. S., perfectly conversational and intellectually intact, was unaware that half her body was immobile and numb. The technical term for it was *anosognosia*.

Right-sided damage, much more than left, leads to a transfiguration of personality. It is these patients who appear in neurological wards with the most floridly bizarre behaviors, their delusions the stuff of literary invention. Take, for instance, Capgras syndrome, in which the patient appears more or less lucid, almost exactly like the person they've always been, except they've become convinced that one person in their life—often the person to whom they've been the closest—has been replaced by an identical imposter. Yes, the imposter looks exactly like their husband, but still, they maintain, it is not their husband.

Or there are patients with somatoparaphrenia, which is a more embellished, more extreme version of anosognosia. Not only do these patients insist that they are not half-paralyzed, they go further: that thing hanging off their left shoulder is not their arm. Yes, they see it, of course they see it! They're not idiots. But it's not theirs. It's their husband's arm. It's the doctor's arm. They don't know whose arm it is, but they'd appreciate it if you could remove it from their bed. What kind of hospital is this where you've got some dead guy's arm lying next to you, hogging the blankets?

The distinction between neurol + psychol illness is totally artificial. Where do you draw the line? Both are always both.

—MARK SOLMS, NOTEBOOKS

What baffled everyone about the case of Mrs. S. was her profound melancholy. She cried all the time. When asked what the matter was, she didn't say, *I'm in a wheelchair for life because I'm half-*

paralyzed and half-blind, what do you think the matter is? Instead, she talked about how much the staff and the other patients hated her, how worthless she was. She was an "oxygen thief," she said to Solms, and she didn't deserve the attention of such a bright young man. She constantly misplaced her things. She lost her glasses. She couldn't find her cigarettes. Twice she attempted suicide, the first time by trying to throw herself down the stairs, and the second by trying to jump out the window. She failed both times because of the very same physical constraints that she wouldn't admit to having.

This was unusual behavior for a patient with damage localized to the right side of her brain. Typically, these patients are much more likely to seem indifferent, bemused, or even slightly euphoric. In fact, their characteristic behavior is so bizarrely unbothered that it serves as the basis of one of the most widely accepted theories of right-hemisphere syndrome; the argument that the left half of the brain produces "positive" emotions, and the right half of the brain produces "negative" emotions, so that when the right side gets damaged, all you have remaining to you are the cheerful machinations of the left. Even then, Solms felt that this idea, in all of its heedless reductionism, was nothing short of absurd.

Solms consulted Mrs. S.'s GP, who'd known her for decades. There was no history of depression. Finding nothing in the neurological literature that illuminated the case, Solms turned to Freud's masterwork, "Mourning and Melancholia."

Here's what's fascinating about "Mourning and Melancholia": even besides Freud's rich, layered treatment of depression itself, it is the very first paper in which Freud grapples with the concept of narcissism. And this, for Solms, was the missing piece, the quality for which he had had no name. But of course it was more than a name, it was the idea, the constellation of features, the particular flavor and dynamic. He suddenly understood. Right-hemisphere patients had this in common: they were all distinctly narcissistic.

Narcissism has become the go-to label of our modern age, easily slapped onto all manner of twenty-first-century behavior, from Internet exhibitionism to the general devaluation of modesty and understatement we might notice all around us. But Freud had a highly specific vision of what the condition actually entailed. Narcissism, for Freud, was deep pathology. On the spectrum of mental health, he considered narcissists much sicker than neurotics. Only the psychotics were more far-gone. Freud believed that true narcissists were unanalyzable. Many in the field would still agree with that assessment. Freud saw narcissism as a profound misunderstanding of one's place in the world, of where one's own self ends and everyone else's begins.

Solms saw that his patients like Mrs. S., with damage to the right side of their brains, were exhibiting the most primitive kinds of defense mechanisms, the tricks we all use in the first years of life, our dogged and doomed attempts to reshape reality according to our infantile desires. Freud describes this stage as "primary narcissism," and it's how everybody begins, unable to relate to the environment as separate from oneself. The defense mechanisms associated with this period of childhood are undeveloped and outlandish; they stand in blatant disregard to reality. Solms was seeing exactly these defense mechanisms in his right-hemisphere patients: reality reshaped according to their desires. They didn't have the paralyzed arm, the guy walking by with the breakfast tray did. The guy in the next bed did. Not them. Whatever the facts, a narcissistic defense seeks its own, self-serving version.

The patients' trenchant solipsism plays out in every aspect of their life, not only regarding their disability, but also in their way of relating to the world around them, and everyone in it. These patients, as Solms would later describe, tend to become withdrawn and childishly self-involved.

"They lose the ability to consider anything from someone else's point of view," Solms would say. Accordingly, they yawn in your face, they pick their nose in the midst of conversation. One woman whipped out a Q-tip as Solms was examining her and proceeded to clean her ears, fixedly studying the results on the cotton swab. Not only was she indifferent to Solms's presence at her bedside, she also did not seem to care that she was being recorded by a video camera positioned three feet from her face.

The problem with these defense mechanisms is that they don't always work. In fact, they always *don't* work. At some point, eventually, they will collapse, because they are straining against reality, and reality will win. The astonishing thing for Solms was how, in the course of a single analytic session, a patient could go from being utterly anosognosic, clueless about his paralysis, to a state of horrified distress—*What am I going to do, Doctor?*—and back again. One patient, whom Solms calls Mr. C., or "the crumpling man," was an engineer in his fifties who had become paralyzed on the left side of his body after a stroke in the right hemisphere. He would barely acknowledge the fact of his left arm, dangling corpselike from his shoulder. In fact, he developed an air of contempt for the limb, the same attitude he displayed towards the people around him. On one occasion, Mr. C. informed Solms that his left hand "was not obeying the orders I am sending it."

Solms came to think of him as the crumpling man because, on several occasions, in the midst of treatment, the patient would abruptly break out into tears, exclaiming: "But what am I going to do if it doesn't recover?" and stare despairingly at his left arm. Then, just as abruptly, he would regain his composure, returning to the cool comportment of a chief executive, tending to business as usual. For Solms, being with patients like Mrs. S. and Mr. C. was like seeing Freudian theory through a magnifying lens. In its outlandish obviousness, it was a cartoon illustration.

Over the years since, Solms has come to believe that these patients reveal the critical role that the right hemisphere plays in normal emotional development. They tell the story of how we acquire the ability to see ourselves in relation to the world around us. The right hemisphere is tied up with our most basic identity, in a way that the left hemisphere is not. Patients with damage on the left side can lose their grip on language, but they normally hold fast to themselves. Right-hemisphere patients, not so.

From birth, the right hemisphere develops at a much slower rate than the left; the right hemisphere takes about five years to catch up, not fully functional until the age of eight. This is approximately the same timeline that psychoanalysts have laid out in describing the psychological progression from "primary narcissism" to "whole object relations," by which they mean the ability to recognize the world around you as it really exists: a mix of good and bad, separate from your own beloved self, outside of your auspices, out of your control. The ability to see the world on its own terms, in its rightful outlines, is a skill we gradually, painfully acquire during childhood, some of us better than others. And it's a skill that depends, according to Solms, on the physical maturation of the right half of our brain.

There is a beautiful logic to this, Solms argues, because the one thing that is commonly accepted about the right half of the brain is that it specializes in spatial processing. Just as the left hemisphere contains the so-called language centers, the right half of the brain enables us to determine our location in space, the capacity that underlies our ability to walk down the street or to fit our hand into a glove. Solms argues that a narcissistic regression is an emotional counterpart for these spatial disruptions: patients can no longer accurately gauge the boundaries between themselves and all others. In right-hemisphere syndrome, both physical and emotional space are redrawn. Such an unexpected merger of neurological development and psychological function is the trademark of Solms's work.

More than a decade after Solms walked into the room of Mrs. S., the famous neurologist Vilayanur Ramachandran published his own thoughts about the curious condition of anosognosia.

"Anosognosia is an extraordinary syndrome about which almost nothing is known," he begins, in his book *Phantoms in the Brain.*

Ramachandran is a behavioral neurologist and an expert on the visual system. He doesn't come from a psychological background. In *Phantoms in the Brain,* he reports on his breakthrough patient, Mrs. Macken, a woman who had a right-sided stroke and became paralyzed on the left side of her body. In his examination, Ramachandran found Mrs. Macken to be "anosognosic for her paralysis"; she reported that her arms were "equally strong" and that she could move both of them normally. But Ramachandran had read of an experiment by an Italian neurologist, named Bisiach, who'd observed that pouring ice cold water in the patient's ear—a fairly routine procedure called caloric stimulation—had the effect of temporarily dispelling the patient's "unawareness." Ramachandran decided to test this out on Mrs. Macken.

"How are you feeling?" he asked her, after pouring the freezing water into her left ear.

"My ear's cold," she said.

"What about your arms? Can you use your arms?"

"No," she said. "My left arm is paralyzed."

"Mrs. Macken," Ramachandran said. "How long have you been paralyzed?"

"Oh, continuously, all these days."

Within twelve hours, however, Mrs. Macken retreated to her anosognosic position, professing to have no memory of her earlier confession, nor any knowledge of the paralysis itself. The cold water had functioned like hypnosis used to in cases of hysteria: while under its spell, the patient could admit to all kinds of things that normally, consciously, she was unable to acknowledge.

It was the case of Mrs. Macken, Ramachandran writes, that introduced to him the possibility that a Freudian mechanism was at work in these right-hemisphere patients. He knew so little about psychoanalysis, but what else could this be if not a good old case of repression?

"It is the vehemence of the denial—not a mere indifference to paralysis—that cries out for an explanation," Ramachandran writes.

He turned to the literature. It was impossible to ignore: the defense mechanisms Freud so elaborately describes were blatantly at work in the right-hemisphere patients Ramachandran was seeing. He recognized denial and repression. Also, reaction formation: the compensatory strategy by which you swear the extreme opposite of what you suspect is actually true. It was common, for instance, for anosognosic patients to make wildly inflated claims about the strength of their left arms, adamant that they could pull off physical feats that they wouldn't have been able to do even if they weren't paralyzed. Ramachandran was astonished to find that Freud might have been onto something.

"When I began this research about five years ago, I had no interest whatsoever in Sigmund Freud," he writes. "And like most of my colleagues, I was very skeptical of his ideas. The entire neuroscience community is deeply suspicious of him because he touted elusive aspects of human nature that ring true but that cannot be empirically tested."

Ramachandran, since warming to Freud, has also warmed to Solms, and sits on the board of the neuropsychoanalytic society. In *Phantoms in the Brain,* he makes an observation that reminds me again of the point that Solms so often emphasizes: the neurological and the psychological are, finally, inseparable.

"What I didn't realize though, when I began these experiments," Ramachandran writes, "was that they would take me right into the heart of human nature. For denial is something we do all our lives, whether we are temporarily ignoring the bills accumulating in our 'to do' tray or defiantly denying the finality and humiliation of death."

8

If I am asked how one becomes a psychoanalyst, I reply:
"By studying one's own dreams."

—SIGMUND FREUD

SHORTLY BEFORE I LEFT FOR SOUTH AFRICA, I had stumbled across an unorthodox headline in the midst of my Solms research: "In Bed with Mark Solms? What a Nightmare! A Reply to Domhoff." The article had been written by the Harvard psychiatrist and dream scientist Allan Hobson, who, it seemed clear, was Solms's most vociferous opponent. Hobson and Solms, I saw, had carried out a furious duet of arguments and counterarguments in endless publications, public appearances, and even in a formal, Oxford-style debate in front of an audience of several hundred in 2006, at the biennial meeting of the Center for Consciousness Studies, in Tucson, Arizona.

I called Allan Hobson. He picked up instantly, interrupting the first ring. "I'm in Boston," he told me. It was as if he'd been waiting for the call.

. . .

To this day, there is no single accepted explanation for why we dream. From the point of view of the brain, the question remains unresolved. What purpose do dreams fulfill? Brain researchers began to seriously engage with the question only in the 1950s. Before then, psychoanalytic theory had been the single arena in which dreams, in all their baffling aspects, had been comprehensively investigated.

Dreams, it had always been thought, are distorted and intensely personal, an unveiling of deeper meanings. Like cryptic prophecies or last dying words, they naturally lend themselves to deciphering. Freud had built psychoanalysis on his theory of dreaming. In *The Interpretation of Dreams,* Freud dissects their hallucinatory shapes, their hidden wishes and attendant anxieties, in order to build a picture of the mind that produces them. For Freud, dreams concealed repressed, unacceptable desires that can surface only while we sleep, and that can only do so in altered form, costumed beyond recognition in order to slip past our internal censor and allow us to continue to sleep, undisturbed. For all the revisions Freud would make throughout his career, working and reworking the role of the id and the ego and later the superego, *The Interpretation of Dreams* stands as the psychoanalytic Bible: all else flows from there.

For scientists concerned with the brain, not the mind, dreams were an unappealing object of query. To study the dreaming brain, it was necessary to rely on sleepy, spaced-out subjects, who were awakened in a lab several times a night and asked to report whether or not they had just been dreaming. (The specific gold-standard phrasing is: "What was just passing through your mind?") It was an inexact procedure at best.

And dreams themselves were a turnoff to most scientists concerned with quantities and chemicals. Ethereal and private, dreams are associated with Freud and Jung, and before them, with mystics and psychics and other questionable figures. It is impossible to observe a dream as one can observe, for instance, the firing of a neuron. To the typical research scientist bustling around his lab, dreams were not a compelling pursuit.

This began to change in Chicago in the 1950s, when an ambitious graduate student, Eugene Aserinsky, and his cranky supervisor, Nathaniel Kleitman, made an interesting observation. Kleitman was running a sleep study, and Aserinsky was charged with the task of monitoring the subjects overnight. He noticed that roughly every ninety minutes, the sleeping subjects would move their eyeballs rapidly back and forth beneath their shut lids—so rapidly that the movement was detectable at a glance. What was this about? There was no mention of this in the literature.

Aserinsky hooked the subjects up to a clunky machine, an early version of an EEG, which measures the waves of electrical activity that the brain produces. The machine had been sitting in the basement of the lab for years. The technology was still in an early incarnation; the printout of a single subject's brain waves over the course of one night consumed half a mile of paper.

Aserinsky and Kleitman (now roused to action by his student's zeal) found that the eyeball movement was only one of a series of activations that occurred on a ninety-minute cycle throughout the night. Still asleep, their subjects would display a sudden flurry of arousal all over their bodies: the EEG waves sped up to alpha and beta, their blood pressure rose, they got erections. Their brains and bodies were in many ways as active in these minutes of sleep as during waking hours. This stage of sleep would become known as "paradoxical sleep" or, more commonly, REM, for Aserinsky's original observation of "rapid eye movement."

Aserinsky had a hunch that this phase of sleep, which lasts

roughly twenty minutes at a time, could have something to do with dreaming, since dreaming would seem to require a great burst of initiative on the part of the brain. Aserinsky assigned a new graduate student, William Dement, the task of testing this hypothesis. Dement stayed in the lab all night, and whenever the EEG machine indicated that a subject had entered REM sleep, Dement woke them up and asked whether they'd been dreaming. He discovered that approximately 80 percent of the time, his subjects woke from REM sleep and reported that they had been dreaming; when he awakened them during other phases of sleep, in fewer than 10 percent of cases did they report the same.

From Dement's data, the conclusion seemed obvious: dreaming was inseparable from REM sleep. The 10 percent of occasions on which people woke up from non-REM sleep and said they'd just been in the midst of a dream was written off as fuzz. It is standard procedure in scientific research to shave off the outliers.

The fact was that having an equation between dreaming and REM sleep was enormously expedient for science. Once dreaming is a quantifiable state, visible on an EEG machine, the roadblock is lifted to studying it scientifically. There is no more ambiguity: when the EEG starts drawing alpha and beta waves, researchers can assume their subjects are dreaming. More important, perhaps, was that an equation between dreaming and REM sleep allowed researchers to study dreaming in animals. No longer did they need a human whom they could wake up and ask: "What was just passing through your mind?" No need. They could hook up any animal—though cats, who tend to sleep more than most, were the favorites—to an EEG and observe their dreaming patterns, alter their brains surgically and chart the consequences. The robust approximately-80-percent-of-the-time relationship between REM sleep and dreaming subtly morphed into a full-blown assumption that the two things were interchangeable, that they were in fact the same thing.

Where Aserinsky and Kleitman had left off, Allan Hobson, two decades later, picked right up again. Hobson took to his own laboratory, where, sticking electrodes into thousands of cats, he further reified the equation between dreaming and REM sleep. Along with his colleague at Harvard, Robert McCarley, Hobson discovered that REM sleep is controlled by something very much like an on-off switch: two groups of neurons, located in the brain stem, alternate in firing, each inhibiting the other, producing the oscillations between REM sleep and non-REM sleep that occur throughout the night.

In a single paragraph in his seminal book, *The Dreaming Brain,* Hobson describes the relationship between the "on" and "off" neurons of REM sleep as "a war of nerves," "an exchange of fire," "a competition," "a contest," "a continuous struggle," and "an underground battle." Hobson's choice of words reflected his belief that what he had found out about the mechanisms of REM equipped him for the central battle of his life: his war on Freud.

To make his case, Hobson emphasized the significance of the location of his famous "on-off switch": the brain stem. The brain stem is the brain's lowliest region, in both senses of the word. It is physically at the base of the brain, connecting between the brain's middle structures and the spinal cord. The brain stem is also the farthest removed from the functions we pride ourselves on, those we consider truly "mental"—our powers of thought, emotional complexity, capacity for consciousness. To look at pictures of the brain stem is to come face-to-face with the indignities of evolution.

Hobson, however, was in ecstasy over the brain stem. It was the love of his life. Nothing suited his purposes more than its unimpressive credentials. Hobson—for reasons I would later learn—had an agenda. For Freud, dreams are driven by intense, primal desires and urges. But Hobson argued that dreams are "motivationally neutral." He himself was not. He was consumed with the purpose of disemboweling psychoanalysis. In this sense, Hobson's career has been the equivalent of lit matches and lighter fluid.

Hobson posited a new theory of dreaming. During REM sleep, as he'd shown, the brain stem flings arousing chemicals upward toward the forebrain and causes a variety of activity there: the cortex coming alive with visual images, sounds, a sense of touch and balance and movement, similar to waking hours, when the activation is mainly caused by stimulation from the outside environment. The difference in dreaming is that the stimulation comes from within. The forebrain, Hobson claimed, now confronted with all these fragments of experience, is forced from sheer, unthinking reflex to patch them together into some kind of unified story line. It thus produces the "synthesis," as Hobson called it, that we experience as a dream.

Hobson's rendition of what goes into a dream did not capture the forebrain at its most flattering angle. The forebrain is supposed to be captain, top dog, of all things mental. It is the seat of every one of our higher mental functions; since Darwin, we have believed that it is the forebrain that most differentiates us from other species. It's what enables language, mathematics, and memories. Anything that fills us with wonder about the capacity of our brains tends to be a comment on the capacity of our forebrains.

But Hobson denigrated the role of the forebrain in making dreams, portraying it as the passive recipient of the brain stem's burblings. Hobson argued that the nightly spectacle of dreaming, the

very phenomena that has captivated humans since antiquity, that
saved the life of Joseph, that inspired the creation of psychoanalysis,
was a simple matter of physiology. It was little more than a gaudy
neuro-chemical fountain that goes on every ninety minutes, regales
its bystanders, and subsides.

And if dreams are made like this, by rote activation and frantically improvised synthesis, how could they possibly correspond
to the complicated creations that Freud had so elaborately parsed?
Obviously, said Hobson, they couldn't.

The whole way to Boston, I listened to radio pundits seizing their
moment, vibrating with news of the economic collapse. It was the
fall of 2008. Lehman Brothers had closed. Cardboard-box busi-
nesses were thriving. And I was en route to Boston to discuss the
history of dreams. The absurdity of this was not lost on me.

Hobson lived in Brookline, an affluent suburb, on a steep hill in
a leafy neighborhood a few blocks from the Brigham and Women's
Hospital. His house was a large Victorian, painted in chic shades
of gray and black. On the front door, a small metal plaque read:
Dr. J. Allan Hobson. After all his tough talk on Solms, I was surprised to see a slightly stooped, white-haired man coming toward
me on the other side of the warbled glass. Hobson moved through
his front hall in stages.

Inside, the rooms were aesthetically detailed, eclectic: Indian
print fabrics slung over sofas, an enormous chair of surreal propor-
tions in the corner. It was academia with a flair. We sat facing each
other in two chairs he had drawn up to his desk.

Within minutes, Hobson was talking about Freud. He gravitated
to the subject. He described his own training as a progressive disil-

lusionment with psychoanalysis. He found out early, he said, that it was "just all made up, speculative philosophy. There is no evidence for it whatsoever."

Freud himself, Hobson says, was a "terrible person." He was "vain," and "he didn't know the difference between science and literature" because "he had a screw loose."

Hobson's voice was virulent. After all these years, Freudianism still infuriated him. I struggled to match up the intensity of his attack with the frail and dusty picture I had of psychoanalysis today, a field constantly defending itself against a chorus of criticism for being expensive, outdated, and unending. What's the point when there's Prozac? Or so the new thinking goes. But Hobson believes that while the institution of psychoanalysis may finally be losing its power, its damage is widespread. Not only is "the whole enterprise of psychiatry poisoned by Freudianism," as he put it to me, but also "the American culture is Freudian wall to wall."

As we sat at his desk, knee to knee, Hobson mentioned a psychiatrist friend who had recently died. "He said he thought we should call ourselves Freudians Anonymous," Hobson said, "because we were like alcoholics trying to deal with the fact that we'd been exposed to this toxic intellect."

"You take such a strong reaction to this," I observed.

Hobson explained that when he went through his medical training, Freudianism was everywhere. There was no respectable alternative. He was never allowed, he said, the airspace to question the dogma. It took him years to be able to lay claim to his own vision.

"I think the way to study the mind is deliberately and patiently and certainly not by means of any Freudian techniques," he said.

I asked Hobson what it means to be in a room with a patient and not to use any "Freudian techniques."

Immediately, he began to tell me about a woman named Iris, a patient he treated for thirty-five years. She was severely anorexic and, when she first arrived at Hobson's office, had already been in a lengthy psychoanalysis, without any discernible improvement.

"When I first met her, she thought everything that was white represented her mother," Hobson said. "The analyst had told her that. Tapioca pudding represented her mother.

"She came to one session with me, and I said, we can't talk about any of that crap. I will see you once a month for thirty minutes and in those thirty minutes you will tell me things that you did in the previous month that made sense. That's all."

I remarked that this seemed a very limited amount of time to spend with a patient.

"She liked me," he continued. "She thought I was vivid and interesting. She hadn't had a menstrual period since she was anorexic. And in the month after she saw me the first time, she had a menstrual period. So what was going on?"

"I don't know. What was going on?" I said.

"She was feeling sexual. I don't know. I suppose."

"So you're saying you inspired that sexuality."

"Well, I think that happened. Should I analyze that?"

"I don't know, should you?"

"No. What this woman needed was menstrual periods. And she had to stop thinking about tapioca pudding."

When I mentioned Mark Solms, I understood the gravity of Hobson's indictment.

"He's a deep Freudian," Hobson said. "Solms is a guardian of Freudian mythology. I think he's very charming. He's just as charming as my stepson in Italy."

"They remind you of each other?" I asked.

"Well, only that he holds these dark thoughts in his mind, and he doesn't tell you about them. Luca doesn't tell you what he's thinking, and he wants to kill you with an axe."

I did not explore this comment, to my lasting regret.

If any one moment can be said to have hurried psychoanalysis along its current underdog's path, it was the publication, in 1977, of Hobson's article, with Robert McCarley, "The Brain as a Dream State Generator: An Activation-Synthesis Hypothesis of the Dream Process." The words "death blow" sometimes surface when psychoanalysts discuss it. Dreams, Hobson was eager to demonstrate, contained no disguised wishes, no latent meaning. Contrary to Freud's vision, the meaning of dreams was exactly what it appears to be. There is no coded significance, no symbols to interpret. "Hobson makes the point that it's such a simple explanation," Solms would tell me. "You don't need any clever Viennese thinking."

Hobson's work provoked a sea change in the scientific study of dreams. He had a polarizing effect: his work, which was based on chemicals and physiology, came to represent "hard" science, good, virile, testable. In her 2004 book, *The Mind at Night,* the journalist Andrea Rock describes how research grants for the study of sleep and dreams drifted in this direction, away from "soft" science— research that was interested in dreams as psychological phenomena. For instance, Rock describes a study by David Foulkes, a research psychologist in Laramie, Wyoming. For years, Foulkes had been testing the same group of children, bringing them in to the lab to sleep overnight a few times a year to see how their development affected the content of their dreams. He found that it wasn't until they were six or seven that the children began to appear as the protagonists in their own dreams, which he hypothesized was linked to their developing sense of agency, a new and important insight in child psychology. After more than ten years of maintaining his longitudinal study, Foulkes lost funding for his research. His, argues Rock, was exactly the type of work made vulnerable by the quest for simple, empirical data above all else.

In Johannesburg at the end of the 1980s, Solms was embarking on his dissertation. Like Freud before him, he had decided to start with dreams. In the crowded neurosurgical ward of Baragwanath Hospital, he was trying to investigate the effects of different patterns of brain damage on dreaming. He knew the accepted wisdom of the day, handed down by Aserinsky, Kleitman, and, later, Hobson: dreaming was the side effect of a fundamentally rote biological process. Nothing more. So how could it be, Solms thought, that he now had a whole collection of patients in whom damage to the pontine brain stem had eliminated their ability to enter into REM sleep— yet done nothing to stop their dreams? According to Hobson, that should be impossible, a contradiction in terms. There should be no dreams without REM.

Solms found that contrary to Hobson's argument, the pontine brain stem was *not* the crucial structure in the formation of dreams. Rather, Solms discovered, it was only damage to another area of the brain entirely, the ventro-mesial frontal white matter, that could bring about the total cessation of dreaming. Indeed, with his longtime collaborator Jaak Panksepp, well known in the world of affective neuroscience, Solms would later term this area of the frontal cortex "the seeking system," or, as Solms also puts it, the "I want" system, because its dopamine-fueled circuitry is the very same structure that contributes to our most basic urges, motives, and desires.

But Solms wasn't quite thirty years old. He was just starting out; Hobson was a giant in the world of sleep and dream research. Solms knew that he had good reason to doubt Hobson's work, but he feared that he did not have enough evidence to persuade the rest of the scientific world. He had only nine cases. He searched the literature, hoping that there had been other reported cases of patients who had ceased to dream after brain damage of this kind.

He found a scattering of reports—one from nineteenth-century France, another from China, in the 1930s. It was something, but it wasn't quite the backup he was hoping for. Then, abruptly: inspiration. In the 1950s, a new surgical procedure was invented to replace the notorious lobotomy. Instead of taking out such a significant portion of patients' frontal lobes, surgeons began to opt for a newer, less radical option: a procedure called the "leucotomy," which involved disconnecting a smaller portion of the frontal white matter. In fact, the leucotomy, Solms remembered, disabled exactly the portion of the brain in which he was interested.

Solms dug up case reports written by neurosurgeons who had performed leucotomies and, following standard medical procedure, tracked their patients after the operations to determine the outcome. In these grim narratives, Solms discovered that, indeed, the patients had lost their ability to dream. Incidentally, the very fact that many of the neurosurgeons had even inquired after their patients' dream lives was a reflection of the era in which they went through their medical training. Modern neurology would not have included the psychoanalytic components that these neurosurgeons, coming up in the 1940s and '50s, were exposed to. This is also, of course, in part why Solms was able to make a unique contribution to dream research: his neurological contemporaries were not disposed toward asking such unserious questions.

It was a crucial finding, and it put Solms on the map. If REM and dreams were, after all, separate mental events, then dreams were restored their significance: it was still possible, indeed imperative, to regard them as psychologically rich and revealing.

And yet, it's an interesting fact that Hobson, too, is smitten with the richness of dream life. He owned and operated a museum in a barn in Vermont, dedicated to dreaming. He often wrote down his own dreams in great detail upon waking and even published a book of them in 2005. (Sample chapter opener: "On Saturday morning, after Lia got up to cook breakfast, I had two incredible dreams, in which I was kissing. In both, my female collaborator was unseen and, in fact, disembodied! I could see only a mouth, wide open in a most lascivious fashion.") Hobson clearly does not believe that "dreams are froth," as Freud summed up the position of his own critics, in 1900, when *The Interpretation of Dreams* had just been published.

For all the arguing, all the airtime, the essence of the disagreement between the two men is, at moments, hard to discern. They are locked into their antagonism like boxers in an embrace. Ultimately, perhaps, the schism is rooted in each man's respective understanding of Freud. For Solms, some of Freud's thoughts on the nature of the "censorship" that the mind applies to the content of our dreams do not stand up today in the light of our more scientifically refined understanding of the dreaming brain. But for Solms, the center still holds: the idea that dreams are driven by intense, primal, desires, wishes, and wants. Whereas for Allan Hobson, any flaw at all in the original dream theory is proof that the whole structure must crumble. "If the dream theory is wrong, you've got to do *everything* over," he told me in Boston.

As my time with Hobson wound down, I mentioned that, as far as I understood it, he and Solms did appear to share common ground. For instance, I said, Solms had conceded that Freud was probably not right when it came to the "disguised censorship" aspect of dreaming. "Make a Xerox, and send me a copy; I'd love to see that," Hobson said. The image of putting a photocopy into the mail reminded me of Hobson's age and fragility. I wondered suddenly to what extent his ongoing vendetta had to do with the simple desire to cling to life.

The next day, Hobson sent me an e-mail. "Solms & Co is as passé as Lehman Brothers," he wrote. "You can quote me on that."

9

IN THE YEAR AFTER MY TRIP TO CAPE TOWN, I would see Solms on most of the weekends he came to New York, the first weekend of every month. Often, we met at Mon Petit Café, a French restaurant on Lexington Avenue where Solms liked to take his meals. We were there, at one of the rickety wooden tables, when Solms produced from his briefcase a plastic bag with a ziplock seal. Inside: five spiral notebooks, in the reporter's notebook style. I knew what they were. I had asked for them. These were the notes Solms had made all throughout the 1990s, the formative years of his professional life.

I thrust the plastic bag into my own, much larger bag, which was in its usual state of disarray, every kind of object—tape recorders, stray batteries, uncapped pens, phone charger, gym clothes—swirling together. An expression of vague alarm crossed Solms's face as he observed the company that his notebooks now kept.

"Listen, I haven't made copies of these, so please be sure not to leave them anywhere they might be destroyed in fire," he said.

Later that night, I poured them out of their plastic bag and onto the floor of my apartment. I squinted at Solms's crowded notations. The notebooks began with Solms at thirty. He'd married Karen Kaplan and moved with her to London, where he was two years into his psychoanalytic training. On the side, he worked as a neuropsychologist at the Royal London Hospital. His handwriting was dense, its own little forest of trees and leaves, strenuous work to decipher. The first thing I noticed as I flipped through the pages was that there were no corrections, no words crossed out, no false starts. I considered the issue of self-doubt. What a luxury to operate with a minimum.

In 1991, Solms, age thirty, was asking himself such questions as: "Could it be that the cerebral representation of the sphincter is somehow directly related to the function of repression / ownership? Probably yes."

Solms began each thought with a designation that clearly belonged to some complex organizational system: 13.IV preceded 15.IV, which divided into the subset b) before leading directly to 22.IV. I would never figure out what these digits referred to. I would spend hours reading Solms's notebooks. There was one theme in particular that haunted these records of his thinking: What, really, can we know?

"It may be that psychological knowledge is the most secure form of knowledge; not the physical. The physical can only become known via the psychological; it is to a large extent an artificial creation, or at least a construction on the basis of incomplete and inaccurate information . . . Also: the problem of observer influence."

In a funny way, I was dealing with a version of this same struggle, trying to understand, through close observation, Solms himself. In this pursuit, I sat with Solms's notebooks like they contained the Code of Hammurabi, like they were a shorthand for the byzantine development of his scientific thinking. Solms's notebooks were laced through with the influences of the psychoanalytic material he was studying. These passages were heavy on the inevitable introspection that comes with that education, the desire to put a grid of meaning onto your own past.

As I know, the child who has to parent itself is at risk in relation to self-destructive trends, negative reactions to success, etc. When it survives (after a long struggle, exhausted by having kept the sun in the sky by day and the moon by night, in the belief that nobody else would do it if it didn't) and due to its over-developed capacities for dealing with reality, it succeeds admirably in something, and then it hears its mother (real mother) expressing her pride, he tries to convert her into the self-protecting object he has had to be for so long; he resents her pleasure, projects the anxiety that probably belongs to her back into her and risks destruction again, in the hope that this time it will be protected from outside, or at least, in order to wipe the smile off the maddening face of the proud mother, when the mother inevitably fails to take over the protection role, the patient assumes it once again and reluctantly and resentfully continues to succeed. (This has implications for Ms. B., except that she, unlike me, does not successfully take on the self-protective form, does not succeed. something else happens. more self-destructions.)

Yet personal reflections like this one were rare: for the most part, Solms was struggling with intellectual and scientific traditions: Kant, Vygotsky, Luria, and, of course, Freud. Or "F," as Solms called him throughout.

In 1993, a moment of optimism: "I really feel that I am beginning to grope towards an answer to the problems which have preoccupied me so. Wittgenstein is right to say that philosophy is a disease of the mind, etc., but I wonder whether he had any knowledge of the possibilities opened up by the discovery of the second sensory surface?"

The second sensory surface occupied much of Solms's thinking, in fact. He used the phrase to refer to internal perceptions, as opposed to the primary sensory surface, which is directed outwards.

In 1995, a spot of self-deprecation: "I am above all and after all just a TRANSLATOR. I translate from physical (neural) science to psychological science, from German to English, and unconscious phantasy to meta psychology (and past to present, psychology to science, etc.)."

But I wondered, was I wrong to trust Solms's self-effacement, his acknowledgment of the limitations of his role? I had grown so accustomed to his confidence, his displays of expertise, his charisma. Maybe, I imagined, he had written this entry in a mood of self-doubt, age thirty-four, new baby son crying in the middle of the night in their small flat in London, keeping everyone awake.

But who could say? As Solms had long understood, "Perception is all that we can ever know with certainty."

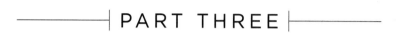

PART THREE

10

IN THE SPRING OF 2010, I am in an apartment on the Upper East Side of Manhattan, surrounded by psychoanalysts. Solms has invited me here to attend a meeting dedicated to the discussion of a few unusual cases, patients who many people would consider to be outside the jurisdiction of the psychoanalytic technique. The patients all share one thing in common: brain damage.

I have returned to this apartment month after month, sitting on a metal folding chair on the edge of the huddle of analysts. The experience is, I imagine, like reading Dickens in the original serial: ongoing story lines, interrupted for weeks at a time, full of vivid characters, perpetually left in suspense.

Outside, the view is airy and blank, the apartment high above the East River, no neighboring buildings to clutter the sky. In one corner of the window frame, I can see the elegant dips of the Triborough Bridge, like tennis bracelets hanging down from slim wrists. Inside, the walls are glossy, the ceiling low, the furniture done in neutrals and glass. Photographs of grandchildren in silver frames cover polished surfaces. There are the bookshelves dotted with the books I have come to understand all New York psychoanalysts are likely to possess: *Three Essays on Sexuality, The Interpretation of Dreams, Civilization and Its Discontents.* Everything the biographer Peter Gay ever wrote about Freud. A sprinkling of the pantheon:

Carl Jung, Melanie Klein, and D. W. Winnicott. A book or two by the contemporary British analyst cum writer Adam Phillips, known for his pith, his wit, and his leather capes. *Man's Search for Meaning.* World War II historians and Hitler experts. The complete works of Paul Auster. A white orchid arcs over the coffee table; month after month, it remains miraculously unchanged.

The apartment belongs to Edith Laufer, a bubbly psychoanalyst who fled Germany as a young woman. Her husband, Jack, snowy-haired, greets us at the door every month dressed in a formal black suit, readily offering his faraway smile. At moments, if I half close my eyes, I can imagine I am in some European city, circa 1930. *The Kleinians have this very disturbing, I think, notion of countertransference as being something the patient does to you. They're moving too far away from Freud's understanding of countertransference as the analyst's own unexamined response to the patient . . .*

But it is, in fact, 2010 and the conversation is new.

Solms had founded this group in 2001. Since then, his ideas had been gaining traction in the wider world: emerging groups of psychoanalysts in London, Rio, Frankfurt, and Cape Town had begun to treat brain-damaged patients according to the model Solms had established in New York, bringing Freudian theory into the room where only neurological fact had previously existed.

On his monthly trips from Cape Town, Solms supervises the progress on East Eighty-Second Street. When he arrives, exactly on time, he is led into the armchair where he will spend the next two hours listening to developments in the group's roster of cases. A porcelain coffee cup is placed into his hand. It is the cue to begin.

Despite all the time I have spent in this apartment, it only dimly occurs to me that directly on the other side of the living room wall, just five feet of bricks and stones separate me from the school I attended for much of my childhood, a strict all-girls school known for its cerebral intensity and blue tunic uniforms, as sexless as cardboard. The view out the window throughout all those years of primary education was almost exactly the same one I am staring at now; yet now I am immersed in a completely different reality, imagining the situations of these patients, and the analysts who treat them.

Every month, the group's discussions are captured by a microphone clipped to Solms's lapel and linked to an elaborate recording device sitting on the glass table.

For the last two years, the analyst Susan Ranawat had been seeing the most severely impaired patient ever treated by this group. He was thirty years old, his name was Theo, and he had been in a car accident during his first year of medical school, an accident that left him in a coma for weeks. When he woke up, it was to a radically altered reality. He had severe global brain damage; he couldn't walk, couldn't talk, couldn't function without around-the-clock care. His mother brought him back to his childhood home, where he had lived ever since. Five years had gone by since the accident, and slowly he had made slight improvements, in the sense that he could scrape together, with enormous effort, a continuous sense of the circumstances around him. He knew who he was and what his day-to-day reality consisted of, and why. His mother, an immigrant to this country, had provided every kind of care for him. Her concern now, five years later, was that he did not seem to have matured emotionally, as if his psychological development had ceased on the day of the accident. It was a sign of her enormous attachment and attentiveness that she had decided to send Theo to psychoanalytic therapy, which otherwise wouldn't have been a course of action natural to their particular family culture. She was willing to try anything that might help her son.

Ranawat had never treated anyone like Theo. When he appeared for their first session, Ranawat realized with a sudden sense of shock that she was imagining her new patient as a child in a stroller, while she and Theo's mother were the grown-ups. Theo, for his part, seemed to have no understanding of what it was he was doing there.

We had heard, over the past months, of Ranawat's growing absorption in the case. But in the beginning, she had had no idea how she was going to proceed. What was she going to do to fill the hour with a person as handicapped as the thirty-year-old man looking out at her from his wheelchair?

After a few sessions with Theo, Ranawat realized that she had to take notes during the session, "otherwise I would just completely lose my bearings." Eventually, Theo asked about the notes, pointing and shrugging to convey his question. Were they for his mother? No, Ranawat told him. "If I don't take notes," she said, "I can't remember what happens in our sessions together." At that, Theo broke into a broad grin. He was enormously pleased to hear that Ranawat had trouble remembering, just like he did.

In those beginning sessions, Theo couldn't retain Ranawat's name from one week to the next; nor was it clear he understood what it was he was doing in a psychoanalyst's office. Gradually, though, he seemed to latch on to the reality of it, called her Doc, greeting her brightly when he appeared at her door. Another shift: Theo, at the beginning, hadn't used proper names or pronouns in his sentences. Ranawat had mentioned, as their time went on, that Theo's narration grew more complete, his grammar expanding to reflect his own role in his sentences. Ranawat made careful records of all his new pronouns, jotting them down and repeating them to the group with a tone of obvious gratification. For her, they were proof that something was happening between them.

On a recent Friday, a woman had slipped in late to Laufer's apartment. She was a visitor to the group, closer to my own age than anyone else there. I recognized her as Heather Berlin, from her various columns in places like *Scientific American.* I was fascinated to see her in this room because Berlin, a research neuroscientist at Mount Sinai, represented a partisan view: she was, from what I knew of her work, not inclined towards psychoanalytic thinking. I had the sudden fantastical idea that she had been called here to intervene. Listening to the presentations, she seemed skeptical, even out of sorts.

After Ranawat had finished reading her latest notes on Theo, Berlin quickly raised her hand. "How can psychoanalysis be effective in such a damaged brain, particularly one where the connectivity is so disrupted?" she asked. Her incredulity was obvious, her word choice pointed. *Connectivity* was a term from another realm, from the world of laboratories and data you can put on a graph and draw lines through. It was a conversational trump card, signaling that hard science had entered the room.

Solms jumped in to respond. "This is the question I've dealt with most in my life. People say to me, 'But don't you realize, you dummy, this patient is brain damaged?' This is your first visit, you have no reason to believe it, but I'm telling you, they really use our help."

On Solms's trail, I had heard a version of this conflict again and again. Solms's skeptics, and there were many, were often asking, in one way or another: What right do either of these two fields have, with their utterly distinct methods and ingredients, to tangle with the other?

"We have an aversion to being with people who look funny and talk funny and act funny and are paralyzed," Solms had said to me. "So to take those patients seriously, to really try and understand: What are they going through? How do they feel? And what is it like to not know what they don't know? *That's* the thing we must do."

For most, if not all, of the psychoanalysts who participate in Solms's group, the brain, in all of its particularities and vulnerabilities, is foreign territory. Even for the few in this room who did go to medical school, it has been decades since they've been confronted with the language and landscape of the human brain. These cases represent the first moment in their careers when they've had to think about, for instance, the right temporal lobe. The neurological factor introduces endless opportunity for ambiguity in an already opaque process. One of the analysts had often worried about the possibility of her patient having a seizure while they were in session. Taking him to the hospital, or moving to physically touch him at all, would fall outside the frame of the psychoanalytic encounter. The group thought carefully about what to advise. Both of these responses would violate the carefully proscribed rules of traditional psychoanalysis, in which the analyst retains a deliberate distance between herself and the patient. Distance is vital for the nature of the work they mean to do together. And this was still psychoanalysis— wasn't it? When I am here, I often hear a version of exactly that question.

. . .

In fact, Solms originally conceived of this treatment work with neurological patients as a preliminary bridge between psychoanalytic ideas and neuroscientific ones. As I had learned, he would hardly be the first to turn to brain damage seeking insight. Many of neuroscience's greatest and most legendary discoveries have tumbled forth from damaged brains. One needn't look past first-year textbooks for proof: inevitably, there will be Phineas Gage, the nineteenth-century railroad worker whose frontal lobe injury—a tamping rod blew straight through his skull—illuminated the brain mechanisms of self-control. And H.M., whose radical surgery wound up providing scientists with the ultimate test case for how the brain organizes different kinds of memory. These men and others like them are iconic in the history of brain research. Today, they continue to be widely written about, their stories retold, the implications resifted. The attention these case studies command suggests that the scientific richness to be found in one person's story can profoundly overshadow data manufactured in a lab. In this sense, Solms's work continues in a long tradition of trying to understand the brain by looking through its cracks. Yet Solms's idea wasn't to wait for the patients to turn up, as H.M. did in a hospital in Connecticut, his hippocampi gone, his amnesia a fait accompli. Rather, Solms decided to seek them out himself and, further, to see what might come from applying to their injuries an unorthodox means of investigation—the psychoanalytic technique. He wanted to figure out, for instance, what it means in brain terms to speak of such concepts as repression, or sublimation, or narcissism, what happens to mental life when the brain gets changed. Hence the tape recorder: strange as it may seem, this room is Solms's laboratory; the stories being told, his data.

. . .

The watery light was beginning to fade as we turned to the last case of the day. David Silvers cleared his throat. I had seen him here before, heard bits and pieces of his case, though we hadn't yet met. Silvers appeared to be in his sixties; a slim man, but not fragile, he had the look of the scrappiest basketball player on the court, the team's surprise ace. He dressed casually and spoke casually; he emitted a quality of warm-spiritedness and immediacy, a total lack of disguise. From previous meetings, I knew that for the last five years, Silvers had been treating a man who could no longer speak. He called his patient Harry.

I was vaguely familiar with the facts of Harry's case. He was young—thirty-eight when he'd had the stroke that would send him, seven years later, into Silvers's office. Before, Harry had worked as a private tutor for high school students in Manhattan; he had been an avid swimmer, often participating in extreme, long-distance competitions. Indeed, he was the embodiment of health and athleticism, until the stroke left him partially paralyzed on the right side of his body, and in possession of less than 5 percent of his former vocabulary. His diagnosis: aphasia. Often seen after a stroke, aphasia affects the brain's speech centers. Harry could still understand and formulate thoughts. The problem, the pathology, lay in his ability to express language. Because of the exact location of the cerebral arteries affected, Harry could no longer get his words out in any medium; his ability to convey meaning, the very essence of any therapeutic process, had been gravely compromised. Yet, for the last four years, he had hobbled to Silvers's office on West Seventy-Fifth Street, where I pictured him clearly, sinewy, defiant, propped up with one hand on his cane, fumbling with the buzzer, making his way inside.

That afternoon on East Eighty-Second Street, Silvers wanted to talk about "laminada," as his patient pronounced it. *Laminada* was one of the only words Harry reliably had at his disposal. A nonsense word, the sounds were strung together, and, Silvers explained, it could stand in for almost anything: *And so on. Whatever. Blah blah blah. Never mind. I told you so.* When Silvers imitated Harry, I was struck by how fluently and affectionately he seemed to do so. It was no half-hearted attempt. His voice changed into an urgent sing-song, not his own. Silvers, small and wiry, spoke in a voice redolent of the Bronx, where he grew up: nasal, punchy, vivacious. When he repeated his patient's labored pronouncements, he was as transformed as an actor stepping into a role.

Most aphasics have their own version of *laminada:* a collection of syllables that for some reason have stuck, emerging as a life raft of sorts, when all other words have vanished. The British neurologist John Hughlings Jackson was the first to note the phenomenon. "Recurring utterances," he called them, observing that they existed in almost every single case of aphasia he encountered. This was England in the 1890s, a decade when aphasia was exactly the disorder that many of the best neurologists were thinking about. They believed that understanding aphasia was going to be the way into understanding the brain.

At that moment, Silvers was concerned about the speech he was scheduled to give at the New York Psychoanalytic Institute the following day, which was, unlike this group meeting, open to the public. Silvers was presenting Harry's case there for the first time, trying to figure out how to condense five years of a highly unusual treatment into a single hour. But what he was most focused on, what he was almost sick with worry over, was the question of *laminada.* He was, he explained, deeply unsure about whether or not to repeat his patient's actual word when he got up in front of the crowd the next day.

"I feel that's like his signature," Silvers said. "I just feel it gives him away a little too personally."

"I agree," one woman said. "It's *him*. It's like a photograph."

"Is there someone with a name close to that in his life?" Solms inquired. The answer, Silvers was pretty sure, was no. But even after four years of therapy, he didn't absolutely know. He couldn't.

"The word has no particular meaning," Silvers said. "So although I could use it, I just feel it's too close to who he really is."

The group murmured its assent. They understood. He mustn't.

Solms waited a bit until everyone else had aired their opinions.

"I think that needs more thought," he finally said. "Because in the case of an aphasic, what he actually says is very important material—it's potentially crucial material." It was clear that Solms was trying to address the concern that any psychoanalyst would have to protect their patient's privacy. "And, if you're worried about revealing the man's identity," Solms continued, "think about what you're already presenting. How many men with right hemiplegia, who are aphasic, who are in psychotherapy, are there at this moment in New York?"

By now I knew that this kind of bold pronouncement from Solms might or might not be true, but that it would have the desired effect: to stop one conversation and begin another.

11

YEARS LATER, when he would tell the story of how he came to be working on a case that could further the bridge between neuroscience and psychoanalysis, David Silvers would begin with 1976. That spring, he was often angry, and he didn't quite understand why. He yelled at the table. He was craving more from his marriage, more attention from his wife. His kids, eleven, eight, and six, were annoying him. A high school history teacher, he was beginning to lose his zest for teaching. He had issues with money. All these concerns were utterly ordinary, he knew. Yet, one night, his eight-year-old, Evan, took up position on the staircase, refusing to go to bed. Silvers, frustrated, began to shout: *Go up, go up!* "He was on the stairs, but he was *not* going up."

Silvers reached for a copy of *The New York Times* and spanked him. Evan ceded the stairs, looking at Silvers as he did so with a sense of grim resignation, his worldview stretching to include the possibility that his father could hit him. It was only a whack with a newspaper, but Silvers was stricken. Almost immediately, he cried. Here, then, was an actual moment, an event, that triggered a voice in his head: *I need to do something differently.*

Maybe therapy. He started to ask around. But more, he wanted to begin to think about really doing things differently, perhaps having a completely new Act Two, outside of the classroom, away from

the chalky lines on the blackboard. He had an instinct: he could
be a therapist, he could be good at this. The thought didn't emerge
from nowhere. He'd gone to medical school as a young man, but
struggled intensely the whole way, unable to get a fix on subjects like
microbiology and pharmacology—but, more importantly, unable
to locate within himself the conviction that he was prepared to take
on that level of responsibility for the lives of others. He'd dropped
out after two years, yet the areas in which he had excelled were psychiatry, neurology, and neuroanatomy. The human mind and brain
were his natural sources of fascination.

As Silvers would later tell me, he soon learned of a teacher in the
English department who was training in psychoanalysis at night,
at the NPAP, the National Psychological Association for Psychoanalysis, an institute on West Thirteenth Street a few blocks away
from all of Silvers's favorite Greenwich Village jazz clubs. The
NPAP was unconventional, even for the 1970s, a golden era for psychoanalysis, Silvers would say, before the very methods of analysis
began to be routinely questioned. Still the prevailing force in clinical practice, psychoanalysis dominated the cultural imagination.
However, by then, many of its most respected training institutes
were insular, impervious to new ideas. In contrast, the NPAP had
been freewheeling from the very moment in 1948 when it opened its
doors.

The institute was founded by the Viennese analyst Theodor
Reik, an émigré who had been a figure of controversy in Europe. As
a young analyst in Vienna, Reik had treated an American patient, a
doctor named Newton Murphy, whom Freud had referred to him.
After several weeks of treatment, Murphy, unhappy with the results,

sued Reik for "quackery." Operating without a medical degree, Reik suddenly found himself at the mercy of the Austrian courts. Freud rescued him, quickly publishing "The Question of Lay Analysis." The paper took only a month to write, but became a passionate argument that a medical degree was not only unnecessary for the practice of psychoanalysis, it was often detrimental. Medical training, Freud argued, interfered with the sensibility most conducive to a good analysis. "As long as I live, I shall balk at having psychoanalysis swallowed by medicine," Freud wrote in a letter to a friend as the lawsuit played out.

The Austrian court ruled in Reik's favor. Twenty years later, having fled a war-torn Europe, Reik was in New York, thwarted once again by the strict regulations of who could be a psychoanalyst. Reik resolved to set his own path. Throughout the 1940s, he gave a series of informal seminars and was known as a thoughtful analyst, trained by Freud. He soon developed a robust following. By 1948, the institute on West Thirteenth Street was already beginning to flourish. Yet it would take fifty years for the NPAP to be accredited by New York State.

For Silvers, entering the field with only a master's degree in education, NPAP's inclusiveness beckoned. Walking into the psychoanalytic offices on Thirteenth Street in 1977, Silvers was gripped by hope. There to get preliminary information, Silvers listened as he was told how to apply, what the training analysis would consist of, and a brief overview of the course work. After half an hour, Silvers took the application and curriculum and placed them in his briefcase. "Thank you," he told the supervisor. "I think you've answered my questions."

"You've got a *lot* of contempt," the supervisor suddenly said, his voice raised to a near shout.

Silvers was bewildered, too stunned to understand the provocation. The moment stayed with him. Finally, he would come to understand that he had inadvertently offended the sensibility of an analyst who was used to announcing the end of every session himself.

"I have been naïve about power most of my life," Silvers says. "Even though I used to be in politics." Back out on Thirteenth Street, Silvers's legs were shaking. He stood, trying to collect himself. "My eye was on this," he recalls. He saw the encounter as an aberration. He had no intention of being deterred.

Earthy, unpretentious, keyed into emotion, Silvers had never wanted anything to do with the corporate world. After his two-year stint at medical school, he'd fallen into teaching and loved it, mostly. Now, almost forty, he'd lately had the disquieting sense that he was avoiding something, that he was "hiding among children," as he'd later phrase it, hiding from the challenge of dealing in the adult world.

When Silvers came in for the initial interview, his interviewer presented him with his very first analytic interpretation: "So you want to be in treatment," he told Silvers, "but you want it to be required—so you don't have to say you need it."

Silvers smiled at the accuracy of the statement.

He did express some doubt. "I've never done any therapy, I'm not a social worker, I'm not sure I'm in the right place here," he admitted.

"You meet thirty kids, five times a day, you don't think you have any background?" he remembers his interviewer responding. "Maybe you have some experience that other people *don't* have, in intense emotional situations about learning, parents, failing, passing, college. Maybe you have a little background."

. . .

New York City, 1977: it was the end of the era of John Lindsay, the Upper East Side Yalie before whom the city had briefly swooned, only to face bankruptcy and soaring crime when he was gone, replaced by the dutiful five-foot-two-inch Abe Beame, a former accountant who would labor to save the city. Silvers would later remember the blackout of that July as a symbol of New York's mood.

Silvers felt as though he were witnessing the decline of New York play out at the public high school where he taught. Born of the progressive open school movement, the school's culture emphasized education as a self-directed enterprise, prizing a student's autonomy and native desire to learn above all else. But Silvers was watching that dream slowly fray, as school politics trumped ideals. Silvers had always understood excellence. From a working-class neighborhood in the shadow of Yankee stadium, he grew up in a world of the children of immigrants who gathered freely every day to play in the streets. For Silvers, the changes he observed at work signaled deterioration, the squandering of a utopian vision.

And so, Silvers launched into his psychoanalytic process, experiencing it as a tonic. His days were suddenly enhanced by a new sense of purpose. On Wednesdays, after teaching from eight to three, he rushed to downtown Manhattan for his psychoanalytic course work. Freud I and Freud II. Dream theory, human development, analytic ethics, the bare bones of analytic training. The NPAP was Freudian, a crucial point for Silvers. He'd had a thing about Freud since he was sixteen years old. At the institute, Silvers encountered a cross-section of worlds: lawyers, artists, professors, social workers. They were, like he was, all seeking some version of the same thing, some way into what they believed would be the deeper truths. The process came with a whole new vocabulary, yet somehow, to Silvers, a familiar one, crystalizing the intuitions that had always occupied his thinking. Between Greenwich Village and Douglaston, he carted the endless reading, titles like *The Fifty-Minute Hour, Envy and Gratitude, The False Self,* and, of course, the Freud. It was the first time he was getting around to finding out what had so ignited him all those years before, when he had picked up a copy of Freud's "Five Lectures on Psychoanalysis," drawn from remarks Freud had made at Clark University, an extraordinarily lucid, almost breezy account of the origins of psychoanalysis.

Three times a week, Silvers left school and drove to Great Neck, where he was undergoing the necessary first step towards becoming an analyst: being analyzed himself. Silvers had chosen his psychoanalyst, Jack Bernstein, from a list the institute gave him. He made his choice for practical reasons—an office near to where Silvers lived, a fee he could manage—and for fanciful ones, too. Bernstein reminded Silvers of his favorite cousin, who was particularly hilarious. He began his analysis with Bernstein assuming that Bernstein would be similarly hilarious. On that score, he was disappointed. "But he wasn't there to tell jokes. And neither was I."

At first, Silvers experienced the process of free association as if he were at a confessional; when he emerged at the end of his hour, it was with a sense of relief, of having unburdened himself of sin. He was unsure, exactly, of what was allowed in the room. Of what exactly one was meant to say out loud. His analyst had a gentle clinical style; he wasn't, as the expression goes, directive, he let the material unfold, he let the patient guide the way.

There was, however, something a bit unusual about Bernstein: he had a second career, as a tax lawyer who consulted with private clients on a part-time basis. Occasionally, the phone would ring dur-

ing their session and Silvers would halt in the middle of whatever
thought had been crossing his lips, waiting as his analyst finished
talking through financial strategy with the person on the other end
of the call.

Silvers, occasionally tentative about raising some line of thinking, something that felt too private or too mundane, would wonder
aloud, is this something we can talk about?

"It's your nickel," his analyst liked to reply.

Actually, they were getting somewhere.

This atmosphere, I like, Silvers thought.

Much of what they talked about that year was anger and
righteousness—and the small moments that opened up onto a
larger insight. Silvers remembers exploding at his wife, Ella, at the
grocery store. "All the important things happen in Waldbaum's. I
picked some dessert off the shelf and said to Ella, let's get this for
the kids. And she said, isn't that really for you? She was right. But I
took that like she picked me off and *got* me. So almost because she
understood that, I lost my temper . . . By the time I reported this
thing, it was almost a joke, but still, it's worth talking about. She
discovered me, and I didn't want to be discovered."

A typical, banal moment in a long, close marriage, yet a lens onto
the challenge of living with someone else's point of view, of chafing
against it, of learning to react differently.

A year went by. One day, sitting in the little room in the back of
his house on Long Island, his three kids shuffled in: the Committee,
as he occasionally thought of them. They had business to address
with him. His daughter spoke for the group. "Dad," she said, "we
want to know: How come you're not Mad Dad anymore?"

These were the words that he remembers more than thirty years
later, because they startled him into the realization that something

was actually happening when he went and lay down on the couch to put words to his thoughts in the presence of Jack Bernstein. His kids' observation gave him the conviction that, whatever its flaws and uncertainties, this was a powerful process, one that could change a person.

Fourteen years of training, of classes at night, of his analysis, of seeing his own patients under supervision. Fourteen years and then he was up for the final examination, which was conducted over the course of a single afternoon. Silvers presented one of his cases to a panel of five examiners. "I wanted this as much as I'd ever wanted anything," he knew.

The committee of examiners passed Silvers that day, but barely. His command of theory was deemed wanting. He later learned that they'd waved him through on a vote of faith. The examiners believed he would continue to develop enough to make up for what he didn't yet possess.

This was how it began. In the usual way. Yet, as it happened, Silvers, at a turning point in his life, was walking into the field of psychoanalysis at a turning point in its own history: the next twenty years would see the advent of a new age, the age of the brain, that, with its onslaught of new discoveries, would force change throughout every arena dealing in human psychology.

But he always adhered to the same core principle, then and now.

"What do you regard as the most important thing in doing this work?" he was asked during his final assessment.

He replied simply. "The patient."

12

WINTER 2013

When David Silvers opens the door for me, it is a frigid day in March; wispy snow still clings to the modest front lawns of the houses on his street. The week before, when I'd called him one evening to see if he would meet with me, he told me right away: "That might be cramping my style." His voice was just as I remembered: raspy, witty, full of life, of aliveness. "You see, I have cancer," he explained. Yet just a moment later, he was consulting his date book and giving me careful directions to his house.

I knew that Silvers had been sick. The last time I saw him, three years before, at Edith Laufer's apartment, he had just been diagnosed. The moment was preserved with absolute clarity in my memory: his slight silhouette rising up off the sofa to announce to the room what his doctors had discovered. Prostate cancer. I had not seen him since.

One week later and I was driving out to the suburb where Silvers lived, in Douglaston, New York, exit 32 off the Long Island Expressway. I was early. I drove around, looking for a coffee shop. The local center of gravity appeared to be a small strip mall with a Starbucks, liquor store, Panera Bread. At lunchtime, I would soon observe, battles were waged at five miles per hour over every last parking space. I had no idea just how many hours I would be spending at the Douglaston Starbucks over the months to come, reading the paper and drinking coffee and looking over my notes from the week before.

For the last three years, I had been on the trail of neuroscience, psychoanalysis, and the frontier zone between them, following Mark Solms deep into his working life and along its many tangents. I had had the chance to see firsthand what it might look like to take on a set of intricate ideas and attempt to modernize and extend them. Yet for all the novel formulations the neuropsychoanalytic enterprise was yielding, and there were many of them, I was increasingly troubled by a single image: the person in the hospital bed. More and more, this particular image came popping into my head, disturbing me, forcing me to question my purposes. Because—and I couldn't escape this question—what would sophisticated neuropsychoanalytic ideas actually mean to such a person, newly paralyzed or mute or blind—what would such a person do with all the theoretical discoveries and hot academic debates swirling around the attempt to unite the brain and the mind? I doubted that such a person would care much about any of it. This was the piece that was still missing for me when I arrived in Douglaston that morning in March, remembering the electric urgency of the cases I'd heard described on East Eighty-Second Street, and hoping, I now realize, that Silvers could answer a great deal more than I yet knew to ask.

I turned off of Little Neck Parkway onto a quiet street, a short cul-de-sac lined with small two-story homes, several of them, Silvers's included, built in the Tudor style, with a distinctly fairy-tale aspect, as if from Hansel and Gretel. At the end of the block, a communal basketball hoop punctuated the dead end.

My impression of Silvers from three years before remained in my mind: a certain curve of the back, a certain dance of the wrists. But now, today, a sick man. It was the first thought I had when he appeared at the door. His hair was thin and white and tufted, not doing much at the moment towards covering his scalp. He was in the midst of weekly chemotherapy shots.

"Treatment is *great*," he said as he led me towards the back of the cozy, carpeted house, away from the chill March weather. "I am not going downhill. My doctor is a real character. 'David,' she says to me. 'You're not going to die from constipation. You're not going to die from being exhausted. You're not going to die from anything right now, so just cool it.'"

We took our seats across from each other in the small den off the dining room. Above Silvers's head, the wall was crowded with photos of children and grandchildren, and with various pieces of grandchild-related paraphernalia, including a collage rendition, in bright Warholian style, of a tub of popcorn, executed by his eleven-year-old granddaughter, "already a qualified artist," Silvers tells me. I settled back in the white leather armchair and glanced around the room: the newest *New Yorker* splayed open on the wall-to-wall carpet; a small bust of Shakespeare on the radiator, next to a framed photograph of Silvers's oldest granddaughter, aged sixteen, a gorgeous, bare-legged gymnast in a black leotard, leaping high in the air, as if flying. In the months to come, I would so often gaze at that photo, drawn to its embodiment of strength and potential.

"Tell me, Mr. Silvers, when Harry showed up to see you for the first time, what did you think he was doing there?" I asked. Silvers paused. He had been at this case for seven years. How to even begin?

"He may have thought we were going to heal his speech. A couple weeks with us, he'll have his speech back," Silvers said. "There can be a lot of disappointment, transference of feeling misled. Not that we misled. But you can understand he could *feel* misled. That we're giving therapy to aphasics, so they're going to speak."

"Even though he's been told by his own doctors that he won't speak again?" I asked.

In fact, in the beginning, Silvers told me, he was far from clear about the implications of Harry's brain damage. Leaving a message for his patient, he heard on the outgoing answering machine recording: "This is Harry Allen." Had Harry forgotten his own last name? Silvers didn't know to what extent the stroke had disrupted not just expression, but thought itself. He was relieved when he learned, soon after, that "Allen" was his patient's middle name.

Harry Allen Strickland grew up in Toronto. His older sister had died years before, when he was thirty. His niece, Alex, lived in Canada, but he rarely spoke with her. A teenager, Alex found it difficult to relate to her uncle, a fact that wounded Harry deeply. *No good no good no good,* Harry would report to Silvers after the rare visit or phone call from her.

Silvers knew Harry did have speech therapists—one in Arizona, where he spent the winter months with his parents, and one in Manhattan, just a few blocks from Silvers's office on West Seventy-Fifth Street. Yet it was impossible for Silvers to know how much help they had been. Silvers understood the temptation to think of improvement in terms of recovery of speech, but this was not the purpose of their psychoanalytic treatment. He would have to remind himself of that.

This was not a person, Silvers quickly saw, who would be likely to turn up in a therapist's office if not for the stroke. Harry was not particularly introspective, nor prone to existential anguish. Had he come to Silvers, on some level, because he was still holding out the hope—however irrational, however impossible—that some magic treatment could restore to him what he had lost? What did he sense might be possible?

"So. Here's the second part of your question, which was asked by Harry. After a few sessions, he said, *You—why—why you?* He realized I'm not going to solve his speech problems." Harry was asking, then, what it was Silvers was hoping to accomplish.

The fact was that Silvers himself harbored (however irrational, however impossible) the vague idea that the treatment *could* restore some language to his patient. The grim facts of Harry's brain damage were spelled out in the medical charts that had been delivered to Silvers in a thick manila envelope before Harry had even appeared at the office. Yet stories of the brain's astonishing resilience were everywhere. Where once it had been axiomatic to believe that, following brain damage, any recovery that was going to happen would happen in the first twelve to eighteen months, more recent neuroscientific research had demonstrated that the brain's "plasticity," its fundamental ability to repair itself, is much greater than once understood.

In his own work with a severely aphasic woman whom he calls Patricia H., Oliver Sacks notes his reasons for faith and optimism, based on the possibility of actual neuronal regrowth and beyond. "At a personal level, there are powers of accommodation: finding new ways or other ways of doing things when the original way is no longer available," he writes. I often returned to Oliver Sacks's work. Bearded, bespectacled, nearly eighty, the British doctor had invented a literary genre all his own, with his many case studies depicting the aberrations of the brain, but always in the most humanistic terms, as a novelist would, with a passionate investment in the details. In fact, in those years, everywhere I turned, it seemed someone was quoting Sacks, reading him, spotting him on the street, or writing him letters, hoping to consult with him about their neurological situation. I came to think of Sacks as a kind of good fairy, insisting upon a vision of the brain as inextricably attached to the person in whose skull it was located, with all the specificity that implied.

Silvers and Harry were doing something, the two of them, low-tech as it was, that as far as Silvers knew had never really been done. For Silvers, beginning the treatment, the sense of possibility was profound. He didn't know to what extent the therapeutic connection he already felt between them could compensate for an injury he knew could never be healed.

Silvers well understood the tools of the psychoanalytic method. First, the simplicity: the weekly (or daily) rhythm, the permission to express. The details matter. One of the most defining features of psychoanalysis is its atmosphere. The feeling in the room. The objects, the colors, the lighting. Time slows. There is a quiet patience, as in certain churches or libraries. It is an hour set apart from the rest of the hours, a chance to look calmly out at your life and to feel, or begin to feel, that there is a wholeness to the enterprise, that it is something more than a frenzied collection of forgotten moments.

Freud said "the fundamental rule" was that the patient give voice to whatever passed through his mind. Well, Harry posed a major challenge to that parameter. Freud also said: "psychoanalysis is a cure through love," a statement which, some claim, has been handed down through history misunderstood, that it is not in the analyst's love for the patient where Freud believed a "cure" could be found, but rather, in the patient's love for the analyst.

It wasn't Silvers's way to research the condition before meeting the patient. But I would soon learn that aphasia had a rich and singular role in the history of neurology. Treating Harry, Silvers thought about a conference he'd gone to at Mount Sinai Hospital, a symposium devoted to the elaborate, intimate communication between mothers and babies, all accomplished outside of formal language. "Speech. Movement, intonation, connotation, frequency, perseveration—there are a lot of ways to communicate," he said. "We're not at that much of a loss from the start if you don't think that way, and I don't."

"It's impossible for anyone to express everything, even everything they'd like to," Silvers read from his first page of case notes. "We're like him in this way. The commonality is we both know what frustration is."

Silvers looked at me suddenly. "So much in there, right?"

"So much," I said.

"And we haven't even started yet."

13

OCTOBER 2006

It was Silvers's colleague Edith Laufer, to whom the apartment on East Eighty-Second Street belonged, who called to tell Silvers she had a patient for him. The two analysts knew each other from the NPAP, the institute at which they had both trained, and with which they both continued to be affiliated. Indeed, Silvers had cultivated a thriving practice since finishing the long training twenty years before, and transitioning from teacher to therapist. He had seen all kinds of people: lawyers, professors, housewives, an engineer, an actor. Now almost seventy, his life was full of family, of grandchildren, and he was beginning to think of retirement.

Meanwhile, Laufer had been making the rounds of neurological support groups all over town, offering the services of her colleagues, psychoanalysts who wanted to work with brain-damaged patients. At Beth Israel Medical Center, she told Silvers, at an aphasia support group, she had found an ideal candidate. "In this group is this guy who's all enthusiastic and he's talking in a limited way but he's full of pep," Silvers would later tell me. "He was the social *macher*. He was the guy who walks around the room and talks to everybody." When Laufer announced that she was there to offer psychoanalytic treatment, "this guy comes hopping over: *yes yes yes, thank you thank you thank you.*"

Laufer thought of Silvers for the treatment right away; and right away, Silvers said yes. Later, he would wonder why. Hadn't he said he would soon retire? Yet now here he was, eager as anything, waiting for his phone to ring. During this period of time, he covered a notebook page with a record of his thoughts. He asked himself if he was taking this case on from a sense of obligation—his tendency— and instantly realized he wasn't. He was invigorated. He couldn't wait to begin.

There was some grandiosity in the mix, he knew. "My reaction to being selected: LOVED IT," he had written at the top of the page. "I'm going to be the best analyst in the world," he told me, looking up from the page. "Watch this."

But more than all of that, Silvers saw that the very idea of taking this on had revitalized him. "Newness. Challenge. My whole practice lit up for me."

On the same page of notes, Silvers scribbled down an admonishment to himself.

"Watch out for friendship," he wrote.

What did he know of this man? "Possible explosive anger," one doctor had written on Harry's medical chart, somewhere along the way. Indeed, Laufer had told Silvers about exactly this propensity. When she had called Harry to figure out the details of the referral, Harry handed the phone off to an aide who was next to him in the room. The aide gave Laufer the wrong information. Instantly, as Laufer listened on the receiver, Harry flew into a rage, shouting nonsensically at the aide, berating him—even without language— until he was breathless. Silvers thought: *Thank God he can express something.*

.   .   .

Silvers understood that the psychoanalytic story of life can be a wonderful one. It is rich in subtext, protective of idiosyncrasies, it is an exploration of the individual: *What does this mean to you?* It is not an injunction: *This is what it should mean to you.* There is room to be eccentric, paradoxical, inconsistent, messy. It doesn't all have to fit on a standardized form. But could psychoanalysis and its techniques, Silvers wondered, really help a person with aphasia?

For Silvers this was uncharted territory. *Aphasia,* which comes from the Greek for "speechless," is not such an uncommon disaster. By some estimates, one in three hundred people will develop aphasia from brain damage, whether by stroke, head injury, tumor, or degenerative disease. It appears in different forms: for Harry, it was Broca's aphasia, also known as expressive aphasia, exactly because it cripples the ability to express meaning, whether in speech, writing, sign language, or Morse code; it is the capacity to get meaning *out* that is almost entirely destroyed. In its more mild forms, expressive aphasia will leave a person fumbling for the right word, and often using the wrong one; in more severe cases, language has essentially vanished, leaving behind mere remnants, a handful of words, often short idioms or profanities. With receptive aphasia, also called Wernicke's aphasia, a different form of the disorder, the result of damage to a different part of the brain, a person can still speak but loses the ability to understand the meanings of words, including their own. Therefore, when they speak, their words are often garbled and incoherent. When both expressive and receptive aphasia strike at once, the result is "global aphasia," and the afflicted person is rendered speechless and bewildered, beyond language. Yet, surprisingly, in these most extreme cases, the implications for intellectual life differ from patient to patient. In an account of the aphasia he suffered after a stroke, the French physiologist Jacques Lordat wrote in the early nineteenth century that though he had lost the ability to understand his own words, and likewise to decode the words that other people addressed to him, still his inner world remained rich with content. "I used to discuss within myself my life work and the studies I loved. Thinking caused me no difficulty whatever . . . My memory for facts, principles, dogmas, abstract ideas, was the same as when I enjoyed good health . . . I had to realize that the inner workings of the mind could dispense with words" Oliver Sacks writes in his book *The Mind's Eye*. Despite such experiences, it is a persistent fact, Sacks points out, that aphasia is often considered, both within medical circles and without, "a sort of ultimate disaster which, in effect, ends a person's inner life as well as their outer life."

Silvers knew he would be dealing with expressive aphasia, yet the clinical details were only vaguely familiar to him. It had been decades since his two years of medical school, decades since he'd given the brain much consideration at all. It might seem odd, but the brain doesn't necessarily come up even when one's career is devoted to understanding the mind.

Finally, the phone rang at Silvers's Douglaston number. He picked it up. He heard: "Okay?" The voice was utterly distinct. Silvers knew at once who it was.

"Is this Harry?" he said. "I've been expecting your call."

"Thank you thank you thank you," Harry said.

Silvers suggested they schedule a time to meet.

There was a pause on Harry's end.

Then: "Mothe—fath—*shit*," Harry said.

14

NOVEMBER 2006

Harry arrived at Silvers's office for his first appointment exactly on time. He was a small man, but with a compact strength, wiry and muscular, a gym buff, despite his extensive handicap. He wore a bulky brace on his right leg, which had, like his right arm, been significantly weakened by the stroke. Nevertheless, he was fastidious about how he presented himself, his clothes carefully considered, expensive-looking jeans, pressed shirt, bronzed skin "like a blueberry," Silvers would later say. In Harry's presentation, Silvers recognized sheer life force, a refusal to fade into the background.

Almost immediately, Harry gestured towards a notepad on the desk. Silvers slid it over to him. On the paper, Harry set down clumps of letters and numbers. He wrote: "AET." Silvers realized Harry was asking whether the psychoanalysis was covered by his insurance policy—Aetna. It was not. Harry wrote down the names of two women, one his mother, Silvers knew, the other he wasn't sure about—a cousin? A sister-in-law? It would take several sessions for Silvers to figure out that the woman whom Harry mentioned, who lived in Minnesota (on his sheet of paper, Harry managed: "MN"), was a second sister, who called every week, to whom he was close. Harry was trying to convey to Silvers what it was he did to fill up his time. He wrote: "Beth, 1–2 mons thurs." Silvers named Beth Israel, where he knew Harry attended an aphasia support group from one to two o'clock, twice a week. Harry gestured towards a newspaper on the desk, pointing out movie times. Indicating, Silvers was pretty sure, that he went to a lot of movies. "What did you see?" Silvers asked. Harry wrote: "casics." Somehow, Silvers seized on the answer. *"Casino Royale?"* Harry, enthused, nodded vigorously.

Harry could muster a scattering of complete words, almost all of them the names of his immediate family members, whom he often invoked in his sessions with Silvers. He used messy, childlike drawings to try to get at more involved stories, descriptions of what he'd been doing. Freud famously likened the work of dream interpretation to decoding a puzzle, "a rebus," as he put it. Silvers was learning the codes, the meanings, the emotional import of Harry's particular set of symbols. A large circle with small circles around it to mean "ate dinner with," a right angle to mean "corner"—to mean, Silvers surmised triumphantly, Cornell Hospital, where Harry saw one of the many, many doctors now in his life. Silvers thought of Harry as his "puzzle man."

Like other patients with Broca's aphasia, Harry could understand what other people said to him, but he couldn't always hear the mistakes in his own words, those words he did manage to get out. He could utter something plainly incorrect and then stare impatiently as Silvers attempted to suss out the intended meaning. *He has no spell check,* Silvers thought.

In their first session, Silvers asked when the stroke had occurred. Harry wrote, "six and three quarters" on the notepad paper. Silvers knew immediately to what the number referred. It had been nearly seven years since Harry's stroke. Silvers noted the accuracy with which Harry produced that number, since all his other numbers, Silvers was swiftly learning, were particularly prone to error, particularly unreliable. Yet it was with painful precision that Harry conjured the exact number of years since his life was turned inside out. Since the stroke, "every *day* is important," Silvers understood.

Besides numbers, pronouns also presented a major challenge for Harry. He might say "you and me," but really mean "my father and I," or "Sam and I." It was up to Silvers to decode these ambiguities, or, at least, to sit with them and absorb some meaning anyway. He was beginning to understand that treating Harry would involve accepting that not everything could be perfectly understood, that some miscommunication and misinterpretation were inevitable. But then, Silvers thought, that's true for every patient, whether or not their brain is damaged. There is an improvisational aspect to all psychoanalytic treatment, an inherent messiness, a gradual, clumsy process of hit-and-miss interpretations, of not knowing, of fumbling in the dark, that still, despite everything, can be of so much value. Was this case really so different?

Silvers had read one of the only cases he knew of that was comparable: a case undertaken and published fifteen years before, by Mark Solms and his wife, Karen Kaplan-Solms. In it, they describe the case of "Mr. J.," a man in his early twenties, who came to Kaplan-Solms after a stroke from a bacterial infection had left him aphasic. Both she and Solms were startled by how immediately and seamlessly he had taken to the "talking cure," the vividness of his communications somehow unimpeded by the absence of fluent speech. For Silvers, this single precedent was an enormous help in grounding him in a certain kind of emotional framework, where he could feel that, despite the unfamiliarity of the situation, he still had his bearings.

Being with Harry, he remembered his fascination with the neurological that he'd first felt as a med school student, five decades before. "'Mothe—fath—*shit*.' So where is that in the brain?" Silvers wondered. "And can there be any reversal?"

"I can just see those neurons going," Silvers would say to me, holding up both hands, inches apart, his fingers pulsing towards each other, but failing to connect.

In his twenty years of practice, Silvers had never been much of a note taker, but right away, at the end of his first session with Harry, he found himself writing down what had occurred in their hour together. He would do this every time they met for the next seven years. Later, he would think about the first session, wondering why it was that he had been chosen, just on the cusp of retirement, to take on something like this, something new and unconventional, something that might be remembered.

15

IN THE NINETEENTH CENTURY, when neurology was just getting up and running, language, and the loss thereof, was regarded as a Rosetta Stone, the portal through which all the vital answers would come. "Aphasia was not only the intellectual and practical center of neurology, but also a focus for scientists and philosophers interested in the field that was to become psychology," writes the neuroscientist Antonio Damasio. It was in 1861 that aphasia earned the field's focus, when the French physician Paul Broca made his historic discovery.

Of course, to someone like the unlucky Monsieur Leborgne, bereft of words in 1861, the prospect of assuming such exulted significance in the history of neurology might not mean much. Leborgne, a man in his fifties, was confined to a hospital ward after a stroke left him able to say only "Tan Tan." Monsieur Tan, as he would soon be known, was not popular on the ward, due to his constant state of agitation, and his terribly short fuse (hallmark traits of Broca's aphasics), but he was the object of curiosity, his condition strangely beguiling to the other patients and doctors around him. He had much he wanted to convey—his expressions and gestures made that clear—but he was stuck with his single monosyllable. At the end of his life, Monsieur Tan was in extremis, suffering a host of ailments, and confined to his bed.

Paul Broca met his new patient on April 11, 1861; on April 18,

Broca stood before the Societé d'Anthropologie de Paris holding the brain of Monsieur Tan in a glass jar for his colleagues to behold. Broca had made what he knew to be a momentous discovery during autopsy: he had located a lesion in the left frontal lobe that he believed was the cause of Monsieur Tan's condition. Broca's phrase would later become famous: "We speak with our left hemisphere," he declared, summing up the essence of his contribution. Never before had language been assigned to one particular part of the brain.

I was surprised when I realized, in the course of my research, that in a very real sense, as he stood there holding up his patient's brain, Broca was the intellectual heir to none other than Franz Gall, notorious even now as the founding father of phrenology.

We see everywhere Gall's legacy in the form of shiny white ceramic heads with various talents and functions mapped out on top, available as tongue-and-cheek decorating objects. What would Gall have made of these alluring, mass-produced toys? He was the rare character to be as infamous in his own lifetime as he has since become, his beliefs about bumps on the skull thoroughly discredited, his reputation as a pseudoscientific racist sealed. Nevertheless, it is impossible to deny the role Gall played, as the nineteenth century began, in propelling forward the study of the brain. By the end of the century, European neurology would be dominated by a belief in "localizationism"—the principle that holds that mental functions can be said to correspond to specific, "localizable" centers in the brain. The connection between localizationist thinking and Gall's own earlier vision is clear. Gall, and the school of phrenology to which his ideas gave way, argued that all human functions and talents, excesses and gifts, could be traced to specific, discrete "organs" within the brain. Gall produced a map of the skull that purported to locate such diverse brain functions as veneration of God, sense of the terrific, murderous instinct, and love of one's offspring (back of the head).

And there it was again, the relationship between mind and brain, or, to put it differently, between the soul and the body. In the seventeenth century, René Descartes had pointed out the tiny pineal gland, positing—though perhaps not entirely seriously—that it was the only conceivable part of the body that could be the "seat of the soul." Descartes helped to further enshrine the division of mind and body, but already, for centuries, no one had made the connection between language and the left hemisphere of the brain. Even throughout the Middle Ages when a substantial amount of new anatomical insight was being compiled from posthumous dissection, "the whole question of localization of mental function was 'suppressed,'" writes Claus Heeschen of the Max Planck Institute for Psycholinguistics, "and even the leading neuroanatomists of that time simply did not dare to make any inferences with respect to localization of the mind."

Gall's theories gained quick popularity in Vienna, but his lectures were soon banned by the Holy Roman Emperor, Franz II, under pressure from the Church, which considered Gall's ideas unacceptably "materialistic." Gall settled in Paris, where he was tolerated, but barely. For all his zaniness, his far-fetched vision and unscientific approach, Gall's work set an important precedent, freeing later scientists to ask whether specific parts of the brain could after all be responsible for specific mental functions.

In France, Paul Broca, working on the brain of Monsieur Tan, seemed to have found an answer to exactly that question. Broca's discovery—which he would substantiate with the autopsies of subsequent patients—pinpointed a spot in the left inferior frontal gyrus, which Broca declared to be *"la faculté du langage articulé,"* as he put it, or "a motor center for words," emphasizing the rather specific function of *expressing* speech, as opposed to *"langage générale,"* which would demand a much more involved neurological story, Broca knew.

Ten years later, in Germany, Carl Wernicke made a follow-up discovery of his own. He identified a site, slightly farther back in the left temporal lobe than Broca's area, the destruction of which, he argued, resulted in the inability to comprehend language. Unlike Broca's patients, people with Wernicke's aphasia retain a wide vocabulary and normal speaking rhythm, but when they speak, their words are nonsensical: they can no longer understand the meaning of what they say or of what is said to them. Wernicke had the idea that the brain must contain a kind of storehouse of "memory images" for language, each word that we encounter over the course of our lifetime leaving an actual trace of itself in our cortex in "a mosaic-like arrangement." Wernicke imagined these memory traces gradually filling up the brain, like money in a bank account, one word per neuron.

Together, Broca and Wernicke's findings seemed to promise that a sweeping vision of the very nature of all brain functioning was at hand. Their obsession was speech. Soon, most of the stars of nineteenth-century neurology would address themselves to the same question, the same lead. Then as now, speech was considered "a model for other functions," notes Paul Eling. And if speech could be understood in localized terms, many neurologists believed, perhaps every other function could too. The very possibility that the brain could be explained with reference to such identifiable, specific centers breathed hope and energy into nineteenth-century neurology, instilling the belief that it might soon be possible to penetrate the most mysterious of the body's organs. This was the allure of the localizationist school: its beautiful simplicity.

Of course, there were nonbelievers, including the great English neurologist John Hughlings Jackson. Jackson pushed back against Broca's position, declaring in 1874 that "to locate the damage which destroys speech and to locate speech are two different things." Jackson believed that the complexity of language could never be pinned to one center or another. "Since speech or words enter into thought, it seems incredible that 'speech' can 'reside' in any limited spot," Jackson wrote. "We speak, not only to tell other people what we think, but also to tell ourselves what we think. Speech is a part of thought."

On the continent, a prominent voice joined the discussion on Jackson's side, decrying localizationist philosophy. That was Sigmund Freud, in his mid-thirties, not yet a psychoanalyst, still a straight-up hard science man, a biologist, engaged in the study of childhood paralyses. He sailed into the fray with a prickly little manifesto called "On Aphasia." Freud believed that the brain is more dynamic than the ideas of localization allowed for. The brain, said Freud, cannot possibly operate as an unrelated collection of parts, each one carrying out its own task, independent of the others. Instead, the brain must be understood as interconnected, each "center" in relation to the others. Later, in the guise of psychoanalyst, Freud used the metaphor of a telescope to capture the dynamism of the mind. It is impossible to say, he wrote, that the image you see when you look into a telescope is "located" on the eyepiece, or the lens, or on any of the internal mirrors. Rather, the image is a result of the ensemble of parts, which together, and only together, are capable of producing it. Freud's position was inspired by Jackson's own: take in the fine points, the moving parts, the full complexity. Freud's belief in the mind's fundamental dynamism, its interconnectedness, began in how he understood the workings of the brain.

But any disorder that eludes understanding for long enough runs the risk of offending its would-be experts. Over the next several decades, the laser beam of attention that had focused on aphasia gradually wandered off. Indeed, the great energy that gripped the brand-new field of neurology had largely dissipated by the end of World War I. The zest, the fever, the hope that bloomed in the last years of the nineteenth century had, it turned out, been the field's great shining moment, a moment that would not come again until the end of the twentieth, when a whole new cast of brain scientists appeared on the scene, believing, as if for the first time, that they were on the cusp of all the answers.

16

FOR SEVEN YEARS, on Wednesday mornings, Silvers and Harry arrived on West Seventy-Fifth Street, at the office Silvers used to see his patients. Silvers rented a second office in the suburbs, near his home, but he knew he couldn't ask Harry to make the trip out of the city. Anyway, it didn't matter. He was thrilled to be there. Silvers knew that he was at the beginning of something extraordinary.

In the course of their first four sessions, with his faltering pen and staccato remarks, Harry gradually laid out the basic facts of his life, as any new patient might. He was forty-five years old. He had never married and lived alone in an apartment in Hell's Kitchen, a section of midtown Manhattan just a block or two west of the Broadway theaters, with their bright marquees and mobs of tourists. For years, he had run his small tutoring company, working with high school kids across the city. Since the stroke, he could no longer work at all. The metal brace on his right leg helped to bolster his mobility; sometimes he used a cane, sometimes not. Sometimes when he arrived for his appointments, he was accompanied by an aide. Sometimes not. But he always arrived on time.

Harry was disciplined and particular. When Silvers arrived for one of their sessions a few minutes late, he found Harry standing at the door, with an annoyed, knowing, lightly scolding expression on his face, arms crossed. "Nah nah nah," he said. His meaning could not have been more clear.

MAY 15, 2007
Early start. Counter transference, 10:45. He was practically in tears. Many appointments this week, not sure of progress. He points up to heaven. He asked about money. I said very little, or nothing. He says WHY. We'll talk about this again later.

Silvers couldn't help but be astonished by Harry's sheer drive to persevere, to get on the subway, to show up at the gym, at speech therapy, at Silvers's office on West Seventy-Fifth Street, to doggedly seek out anything that might help him live better, even just a little better. Indeed, the persistence of this kind of self-possession in the face of neurological damage is a notable fact about people with Broca's aphasia. Mark Solms, who has observed hundreds of cases of aphasia, had written extensively on the subject. In his book *Clinical Studies in Neuro-Psychoanalysis,* Solms and his wife and coauthor, Karen Kaplan-Solms, describe the profound differences they have observed working with patients who have damage to the left half of their brain, like Harry, versus those whose injury has struck on the right.

Solms conceives of the distinction in terms of "ego intactness." Patients with left-side damage are afflicted with all kinds of losses and deficits, and yet somehow they are able to retain some basic essence, call it their ego, their personality, their preferences, their passions—whatever name you apply to that most basic core self, left-side damage alone will not dispel it. It is when the injury strikes the right half of the brain that these foundational features become more vulnerable to distortion, even erasure. When I went with

Solms on his rounds in the neurology ward of Groote Schuur, I had the chance to see for myself what it is to encounter a patient with a certain kind of right-hemisphere injury. The quality has shifted: they are no longer fully with you, dealing in your reality, or you in theirs.

JUNE 11, 2007

He was angry at the niece when she was young and didn't relate to him. Angry at me for not understanding him so quickly . . . He had a doctor's appointment . . . Very discouraged. He doesn't have much to do. He'll often say, not much, not much. I said, don't worry about it, we'll trip over something. He points up. Meaning, I want to go there, I want to die already.

One day, early in their treatment, Harry arrived at Silvers's office with a machine, similar to an iPad, which he was eager to display. The gadget, Silvers understood, stored information digitally, like Harry's medical history to show to new doctors, or a list of food for when he was ordering at a restaurant. "Let's say he goes into a restaurant by himself. He can't speak, but he can order an iced tea and a sandwich," Silvers would later explain to me. "And if there are further questions, he can elaborate. You want some mustard on that? Okay or not okay." Any gadget, any tool, that made living independently even slightly easier was of crucial importance, Silvers understood. Yet when Harry brought out the device to show it to Silvers, it wasn't working. It wouldn't turn on. He fumbled with it in his clumsy grasp. No luck. He passed it over to Silvers, who fumbled with it some more. Silvers was suddenly desperate that it turn on, that he be able to make it work. He became frantic. He told Harry he'd be right back and rushed out to Radio Shack four blocks away to search for batteries. He had no idea what kind of batteries were required. Nor did he know how to open up the device to insert whatever batteries might fit.

By the time Silvers got back to his office, half the session had gone by. Harry was sitting in his chair, surprised and incredulous and a little bit amused at the spectacle of his harried analyst. He looked at Silvers and shrugged, the expression on his face immediately legible. *Why why why?*

17

SUMMER 2007

Silvers had a terrible dream during the first year he was seeing Harry. He jotted it down. With a blue crayon, he drew a man in a rocket ship.

"He's an experimental animal and we're using him like a guinea pig, shooting him into outer space, like the Russians," Silvers told me when we discovered the drawing tucked away with the rest of his notes on Harry. "He can't speak, and I can. It's survivor guilt. It's: he doesn't have what I have and I'm using him. One thing he can't speak, now you're using him? Furthering yourself as a big analyst?"

Silvers had forgotten the dream until we stumbled on the drawing, but the fact was, a certain kind of ambivalence persisted in Silvers's relationship to the treatment, off and on, throughout the seven years it lasted. On the one hand, Silvers was passionately attached to the case; on the other, its very unfamiliarity could cause him to feel that it could be lost at any moment. Harry might sit for long stretches without saying a word, without making a note, as if to say, now what? The process was granular and maddeningly slow. At times, the very possibility of progress seemed like a fantasy.

JULY 9, 2007

Why do I do this, to what end. Why do I do this work? It
was a collaborative effort, I established that right away. He can
help us to help other people deal with this problem. And that to
a guy who had been a functioning person is a very calming,
relieving idea.

With Harry, the work continued, the questions multiplied.
"Here, I'm getting an education. After all, we're psychoanalysts,
we're not neurologists," Silvers said. "You come in as an ignoramus
in this field. But now I know, the speech and the mobility, that's his
difficulty, goes along with the Broca's, and the injury to the cerebral artery that is the starting point of the stroke is directly related
to these disabilities. So that's the anatomical, biological if you will.
Now I go to work. Can we be of any help psychoanalytically? Well,
how the hell are you going to get into discussions of his deep dark
past—he can't say four words in a row in a sentence. So that's the
question."

Harry at forty-five lived a narrow, circumscribed life: lots of
movies. Work-outs. Meetings at an aphasia support group downtown with his friend Sam—*"good people good people good people."*
Dancing, to some extent, dancing in his chair. Sam took him.
Harry loved to dance. Hearing this, Silvers briefly made to demonstrate his own dance moves. Harry waved him away dismis-
sively. Winters in Arizona with his elderly parents, who wanted
him there all year round, fearing he could no longer look after
himself.

Harry was irritated by his parents' intrusions, but he was now,
as well, dependent on them. Talking about his parents one day, he
pointed up at the ceiling, then at himself, then up at the ceiling

again. Silvers understood. *If they die, I die.* Harry had made the gesture before. Pointing at his crippled right leg, he shrugged. But then he gestured towards his mouth, and pointed up at the ceiling. The paralysis, he could live with, he was conveying to Silvers. It was the loss of speech that killed him. And underneath, it was as if he were trapped, the same man as always, with little recourse for crossing the gap that now lay between him and everyone else. A few years before he had traveled through Europe with a lover. Now, he could describe that trip only as "Fr," "Ba," and "M." France, Barcelona, and Madrid, Silvers finally surmised. Now, Harry was alone.

Quickly, Silvers and I are into our routine. Once a week, I borrow my father's car and make the trip up the Long Island Expressway. Occasionally I run into Silvers's wife, Ella, forever on the move, coming and going, conveying an intensity of purpose and a seemingly unquenchable store of kinetic energy. At seventy-three, she volunteers every week at Planned Parenthood, teaches writing at a local community college, and works out every day. She has the vitality and the body of a much younger woman. When I look up from the white leather armchair, she might be arriving in her exercise clothes or leaving in her motorcycle boots. She radiates empathy, modesty, and insight. Somehow she is deeply familiar, yet she maintains a certain distance. When I ask if I can interview her about her own sense of her husband's long case, the conversation becomes awkward. She agrees, reluctantly, but calls me a few days later to cancel. We do not reschedule. I discover that I admire her even more for her disinclination to speak to a journalist.

. . .

For our sessions together, Silvers and I get ritualistic. He takes out his thick Harry file and places it beside him on the sofa. I turn on my tape recorder and position it near him on the radiator. Then I scoot a little red footstool over to where I can peer at the notes Silvers holds in his lap, the bright light of the lamp next to him shining on his still-thin hair. Week by week, we work in order, beginning from the earliest sessions, scrutinizing the letters and symbols Harry had drawn on his piece of yellow legal notebook paper, trying to understand what Harry had been trying to say, as if to simulate the process as Silvers had originally experienced it: confusion, with occasional toeholds. Once we've given Harry's notes our best efforts, Silvers flips over the paper to read aloud from his own notes, stapled to the back, written after Harry had left. Often, Silvers's post-session notes illuminate some, but not all, of Harry's intended meaning.

Early in the summer, I crane my neck as we study a particularly sparse page, written by Harry on July 30, 2007.

Franke
Can
Hous
Chris

And, scrawled lower on the page, "Irw," with the number 52 floating somewhere nearby.

"I think you said something about 'Frank' last time that was correct," Silvers says, referring to a friend of Harry's who had appeared in the case notes we'd gone through the week before. Yet that idea doesn't quite click in the context of the page we have before us now, with its "Franke" at the top of the list, and we're both silent, staring at the collection of words and numbers.

"Or I wonder if it's a street?" I say suddenly, looking at Harry's list of names.

"Christopher Street, Canal Street, right right! That's very logical," Silvers says.

"Oh—Houston!" I add. Suddenly we know: the four items at the top of the page are a sequence of subway stops, delineating Harry's route from one place to the next.

"Man, you're good at this. You *can't* get better than me—that's out," Silvers says.

"I think there's no chance of that," I say. "But that's my neighborhood, so you see I have the advantage. It's funny that he does the same thing as he does with numbers, needing to spell out the whole sequence to get anywhere."

"*Right.* The sequence helps him. And neurologically you feel that someday they're going to say, he's a sequence guy, or for him the sequence capacity enabled him to count, to locate, to describe. Another person avoids sequences, you know what I mean, you don't know how their brain is organized. For him, sequences help."

I look up from the pages to see Ella through the window, standing in their tidy, verdant garden, spray-painting white lawn furniture whiter. A thousand tiny specks rise up around her in the wavy afternoon heat as she goes. Unable to extract any more meaning from Harry's page, we turn to Silvers's notes. He reads them out loud with characteristic exuberance. "He made a match! His friend Max with the daughter of his parents' friend. He put it together fast, and I understood him right away."

Silvers sets the paper down again. "Now how the hell did he

get that story across to me?" Silvers searches his memory and then seems to recall the moment, Harry explaining that he had put into place a romance between two family friends.

"'We each congratulated ourselves on being able to understand his explanation and we laughed,'" Silvers read, returning to the notes.

"'But we reached a point when sadness was on his face and on my mind, after we communicated the reality of not being able to speak. Like: we did this, but we did this in spite of the fact that he couldn't speak. Alex—that's his niece—came to visit with his parents and the four of them got together at his place and he made chicken dinner for them. He had felt more togetherness with Alex, but not sure after this, would she go back to not communicating with him. He was concerned that she would slip back. I felt he was saying, she'll go back and I won't communicate with my niece again. He came himself, no aide. So he can get on a subway. I was worried that he wouldn't be able to. Then he said, thank you, thank you. For many things.'

"Sometimes he'll give me sixteen different clues as to what he's trying to tell me," Silvers tells me. "It's very frustrating. He goes: *Da-da-da*. He'll give me a few letters and a word and a sound and I'm not getting it, and he gets pissed off. He goes: *Why why why?* How many times do I have to tell you before you get it? He's telling me stuff that's very obscure, but the effort he's making is so tremendous that he's saying: Asshole, why don't you get it already? And when I finally get it: *Why why why?* What took you so long?"

A striking fact about Silvers: he is a natural mimic. When he describes Harry in session, I notice right away he is not merely quoting his patient, but channeling him, stepping into the voice, the gestures, the effort behind the truncated speech. Right away, I wonder about the scrupulous boundaries of the psychoanalytic situation. Was this case so special to him that Silvers had let go of the rules? To what extent *should* the rules be renegotiated?

> 9.24. 2007
> *His schedule. Many appointments, but he said, he's not*
> *better. In other words, no good no good. In other words, he went*
> *to a lot of places and he wasn't so happy with what the results*
> *were. He says Mother, as if she'll be hurt by him dying, or she'll*
> *die, and so will he . . . His shoulder seems a lot better. The machine*
> *is being fixed . . . We talked about loss of relationships and*
> *speech.*

Since the stroke, Harry could no longer work; therefore he had no income, other than what his parents sent him. Silvers decided he would charge only a small fee, one that wouldn't require involving Harry's parents. Harry pulled the bills out of his wallet with enormous difficulty—or reluctance? It was impossible for Silvers to tell. "It's hard to pull money out of your wallet when one of your hands is crippled," Silvers would tell me. Harry's insurance policy didn't cover psychoanalysis. "He may have thought he shouldn't be paying me at all," Silvers said. Yet the payment, however nominal, was a crucial aspect of the therapist-patient dynamic, professionalizing the endeavor, preserving the boundaries.

Early in their time together came another moment that would stay with Silvers for years, a moment that would become, for him, emblematic. It was prompted by Harry's shirt, emblazoned with the logo for the New York Nets.

"This therapy is never going to work," Silvers told him. "I'm a Knicks fan. You go to games?"

"Yes yes yes," Harry responded. And then, with his hands, he invited Silvers to come with him.

Silvers, like many in his profession, was often offered things by his patients, tickets to games, medical referrals, and he was used to turning them down. Yet in this case, it was all too apparent how deeply Harry longed for companionship, how much the process of communication they had begun had whetted his desire for closeness. In New York, Harry had few friends. He had Sam, he had a sister on the phone, and he had various groups to which he belonged, but that was, as far as Silvers could discern, largely the extent of regular, personal interaction in Harry's life. Harry was not morose, but he was lonely, and his loneliness became palpable that day as he thought about watching a basketball game with one of the few people who could understand—or would try to—what it was he wanted to say.

Gently, Silvers said, "That's so nice of you, man, I'd love to. On the other hand, it would change our relationship. So it wouldn't be about dealing with the position you're in. It would become about the Nets and the Knicks and the 76ers and everything else. But I'm here for this. And I think you're here for this too."

Silvers could see Harry's disappointment as he sank back in his chair, retreating into his habitual isolation. So Silvers went through it a couple more times, in different ways. The need to remain within the bounds of professionalism. The need to maintain the therapeutic setting. Knowing his own attraction to his patient, Silvers had to keep his distance.

Harry listened. "Okay okay okay. Okay."

"You could see him literally filtering this through a filter that says: 'He's right but I wanted to and now I have to give up that fantasy,'" Silvers said. As the session time ran down, Silvers saw that Harry remained in a state of bruised withdrawal.

"I see that look on your face," Silvers said.

"No no no," Harry said glumly. He paused. "Okay okay, okay." He began picking up speed. "Good good good."

"See, that's why this is such an interesting case," Silvers told me. "There are people who wouldn't have expressed that in years. They'd tell themselves: 'I shouldn't be disappointed. After all, he's a professional.' With well-spoken, articulate people, sometimes speech is in the way of getting to the feelings."

With Harry, Silvers continued, "his feelings are powerful and if I recognize them and appreciate them, it stabilizes his world." This recognition, growing deeper, this capacity to name feelings that Harry could not, was one of the therapy's most central goals. Even just the attempt to hear Harry seemed to reassure him. Almost no one would do that anymore.

Still musing all these years later on the basketball incident and what it revealed about their growing rapport, Silvers told me, "In my own way, I was looking in the mirror, figuratively, and thinking, to what extent will we have homosexual feelings? They're not disallowed."

"Does that come up with every male patient?" I asked.

"You know something, I'm going to say yes. But only because in various degrees, especially in our culture, men are very afraid of that. I went through it in my own analysis, I have all these feelings for this guy, does that make me gay? I think there's a reaction to loving another man, by men, that makes many men panic. I mean deep."

.   .   .

The stroke that capsized the left cerebral artery in Harry's brain, that crippled his right arm and leg and scattered his words, left behind an unpredictable store of language. Once, in an early session with Harry, Silvers was taking down some information, and he noticed that the pad he was using had French numbers along the top, manufactured by a French company. *"Un deux trois,"* he read aloud, unthinkingly.

"Quatre cinq," Harry responded.

"Clear as a bell!" Silvers tells me. "It's so interesting what sticks."

Like any psychoanalytic therapy, this one was going to be improvisational, hit and miss, but the very effort at understanding, with all its limitations, was of worth. There was grandeur in the very effort to know. A larger question, for the future, for both therapists and scientists: Did salvaged human connection have any physiological impact? Was it, to any degree, curative? This was the sort of discussion that inspired Mark Solms. Once in a while, in sessions with Harry, a full sentence would emerge, like: "I don't go there."

"Well, that's a lot," Silvers says. "So in tiny, tiny ways, maybe we do have recovery of a little bit of speech." Yet it wasn't his aim to fix Harry neurologically. He knew he couldn't. "I felt like that would be knocking on a door that couldn't open," Silvers would tell me.

10.22.2007

It was a very up meeting because we were talking about movies and travel. He looks good, didn't need a cane to walk into the office. Support in the treatment. What does it mean in the transference that I'm supportive? . . . There's a remarkable absence of content about the father. The absent father's a common theme in all these things . . . I felt his speech was improved. More connection between words. When he talked about his sister, I got a little more phraseology than I did with others. I think he felt support because she calls him every week. Maybe in some way, it helps him to have more connection in his verbal expressions.

18

SPRING 2013

"Actually, there's an article in *The New York Times* today, it's fantastic—did you see it? It's about the mouse brain," Silvers was saying, looking revved up on the sofa.

Through the window, I noticed the garden had come into bloom. My eye gravitated to the new green grass. It had been a long winter. Silvers fumbled through the pile of papers next to him and retrieved the article he'd clipped out to show me. The piece, titled "Brains as Clear as Jell-O for Scientists to Explore," was about a recent advance in neuroscientific technology that had allowed scientists to make a mouse brain transparent, exposing the neurons and networks inside. Beneath the headline, a photograph showed a neon green silhouette of a brain, glowing like a Rothko.

"My feeling is that the brain is a switchboard of *such* magnificence," Silvers said. "It may not be able to hold as many numbers as a computer, but it can associate the color of that bicycle with the fight I had with my father when I was two. A computer doesn't do that, but the brain does—because of the meaning."

Silvers pointed again to the *Times* piece.

"So what I'm thinking as I read this: What's the meaning of these neurons? We're gonna come back to meaning whether we like it or not, scientists. The blood supply is cut off by the stroke. What does that mean to a human being? The psychoanalytic content is the meaning of the injury. We can't escape meaning."

The newspaper fluttered as Silvers made his point.

"They're getting closer. I'll tell 'em when they got it!"

Satisfied, he flicked the paper away.

I was aware that Silvers's clinical style did not strictly conform to what is considered "analytic behavior," a mode of conduct Janet Malcolm captures in her book *Psychoanalysis: The Impossible Profession.*

"The analyst," Malcolm writes, "does not give advice, he does not talk about himself, he does not let himself be provoked or drawn into discussions of abstract subjects, he does not answer questions about his family or his political preferences, he does not show like or dislike of the patient, or approval or disapproval of his actions. His behavior toward the patient is as neutral, mild, colorless, self-effacing, uninterfering, and undemanding as he is able to make it."

And not only with Harry, though with Harry it was surely true, Silvers, I could see, was infinitely more familiar, personal, complimentary, suggestive, directive, self-revealing, and so on, than any of the more rigid strictures of psychoanalytic technique would like him to be. In fact, I suspected, Silvers's approach might well disqualify him from being considered truly psychoanalytic by many, if not most, if not all, of the purists. And yet, no one was more outlandishly "unpsychoanalytic" than Freud himself, who liked to chat with his patients in the waiting room, who let his little lion dog Yofi roam freely through the office as his patients free-associated, who would from time to time analyze friends on the street as they walked together to the theater. Yet even for someone like Silvers, who was not invested in the doctrinaire, the nagging question "Is this psychoanalysis?" would occasionally surface and exert an anxious-making and dampening effect, like a school principle sticking her head through the door of an unruly classroom. It is also true, of course, that to a great extent all psychoanalysts often or even always struggle with the question of whether they are doing psychoanalysis. As the psychoanalyst, philosopher, and writer Jonathan Lear writes in his book, *Therapeutic Action:* "Psychoanalysis is in part constituted by an ongoing debate about what psychoanalysis is. We may not know all the answers, but we constantly live with a sense of a boundary condition: *this* would betray the analysis."

Outwardly, Silvers is unbothered by the breaches of psychoanalytic dogma he has committed along the way. Often, as Harry would leave their sessions, he extended his hand—his good hand—to shake Silvers's own. When he did, Silvers readily grasped it. Silvers knew that "there are probably whole chapters written in journals about not shaking your patients' hands," as he said to me. "But this man has so few ways to connect. Let's connect."

When, after one session, he saw Harry struggling to zip up his coat, his bad hand clenched in a clumsy knot, Silvers reached over and did it for him. Silvers was well aware of the implications. "I could be zipping his fly, understand?" was how he put it to me. And yet it was winter, and his only thought was not to let his patient out into the cold with his jacket open. With another patient, Silvers might have asked in the next session what it had meant to them to have their analyst do up their zipper. With Harry, he hesitated, knowing that this patient would likely wave away the question, regarding it as trivial or irrelevant.

"Don't worry, fourteen police cars are not going to surround the institute and come in and get me," Silvers said, looking at me with an arch expression. "You know, the psychoanalytic police?"

Actually, I did know the psychoanalytic police. I had met them in London. I didn't say it to Silvers, but a part of me was inclined to admire their philosophy of reticence on the subject of what one should or should not do.

One day, Harry arrived at Silvers's office looking strapping, robust, lit up. In a fizz of excitement, he managed to convey to Silvers that he had met someone—or rather seen someone, maybe, Silvers couldn't quite tell—at the gym, someone he was interested in.

Silvers chimed in immediately. "Are you going to talk to her? You should really talk to her."

"I do suggestions, which are sometimes frowned upon by the psychoanalytic police," he told me.

"Did you ever wonder how you were going to fill the hour?" I asked Silvers one day. The question was personal: full of self-doubt, I was often fearful of silence, of failing to come up with the next thing to say.

"Yes, because there is boredom, direct boredom. On his part. Like, *I dunno, not much . . . Nothin'* . . . It could go like that. You could get a little nervous about it. But I'll be patient with that. I'll wait. Or then I'll say something like, did you see Sam this week?"

Silvers told me that the specific texture of their boredom was a feeling of boredom being imposed, like marching orders: we will be bored today. "It's like he's trying to transmit to me that we are going to do nothing," Silvers said. "I'm an inveterate school-goer, I can handle being bored, but that's not the point. I want to *get* somewhere with these forty-five minutes."

He was intent on making use of every available moment with Harry, determined to get somewhere—but where? Somewhere else.

The movement itself was vital. The translating of Harry's "casics" into *"Casino Royale,"* when Silvers asked if he'd seen any movies, "butt" into Butterball chicken into the knowledge that Harry had made dinner for his family the last time they all came to town, a point of pride. Small, mundane, concrete details. Didn't matter what kind of details. What mattered was the communication itself.

"I didn't care where it went, as long as it went. I believe in free association. Even Eric Kandel's work shows that association is not up to our little language to make the decisions about what comes next. Those neurons hit each other. It's not because we learn grammar— it's because the way the brain is structured that we can learn grammar. *So let him teach me his grammar.*"

Perhaps it wasn't an accident that Silvers seized upon the work of Kandel, of all the possible neuroscientists he could have cited. Kandel had an unusual fact in his background: he had started off his career with the intention of becoming a psychoanalyst, completed his psychiatric training, had an analysis, and, though he decided to steer off in the direction of the hard sciences, he has continued all his life to advocate for the power of the psychoanalytic technique— and, as well, to urge the psychoanalytic profession in a more biological direction. I had heard him speak on the subject at more than one conference. In his influential essay "Psychotherapy and the Single Synapse," Kandel writes of his belief, or his "delusional optimism," as he says, that "biology can transform psychoanalysis into a scientifically grounded discipline." Yet I was struck by the terms of Kandel's vision. For, notably, he did not believe that the biological could replace or supplant the psychological. "It does not produce richer paradigms," Kandel writes of the potential of neurobiology. Indeed, he continues, "psychology and psychoanalysis are potentially deeper in content."

Talked about terminations. Didn't get an answer to two questions. Why, why now. Why would a person terminate? Any patient might say, I don't have the money. I think he said the word pay pay pay. He may have been a little pissed off at having to pay anything . . . He seems to want to stop like someone who doesn't get or appreciate the possibility of deeper work. Wants a friendship with me . . . Disappointment. I suggested appointments in September. He was not happy about that. He took my appointment book! And he said, in his way, August fourth. None of this September stuff. My previous anxiety re: his leaving is acting on my negative countertransference . . . Very little money, more time and energy than I had thought, not much analytic work in a sense. Maybe I was feeling guilty or incompetent . . . We hugged. His deep appreciation. More pills every day. Breakfast lunch and dinner.

He had been seeing Harry for several months when Silvers wrote the word "depression" in his notes. "I finally had to give some name to the fact that he's alone and angry and he's depressed about it," Silvers told me. Harry's mood, in session, could trip into irritation, frustration, impatience with Silvers, boredom with the very endeavor. And less often, someplace perhaps closer to the truth: tearfulness would come on from time to time. Describing all the doctor's appointments he had had the week before, Harry started to gesture. So many appointments, so much effort, and for what? To what end? Often the subject of Harry's former working life would make him cry. Silvers understood his tears to be an expression of grief over the loss of purpose, the feeling of having been made futile right in the midst of young adulthood. In a sense, it should seem obvious that Harry would be desolate, teary, hopeless, and yet I found that it wasn't. Whenever Silvers came across "tears" in his session notes, I was always momentarily surprised, because the person Silvers had conjured up for me, the vision he had passed along, was not nearly the tragic figure the facts alone suggested. Any assumptions I'd had at the beginning of the process—hearing about the case in Edith Laufer's apartment, and imagining this man as a helpless, crippled shell—vanished so quickly I didn't realize they'd gone or, rather, could barely remember having had them.

In the fall of 2007, one year into the treatment, Silvers was talking the case over with Mark Solms.

"These patients, they're described in the behavioral neurology textbooks as being prone to 'catastrophic reactions,' and really wrenchingly sob. Is that what you mean when you say 'cry'?" Solms asked.

"Not quite," Silvers said. "Some tears come. Then he takes a breath and recovers."

"I've seen many aphasic patients, and I've never seen these 'catastrophic reactions,'" Solms said. "Us people, who deal in feelings, we don't see this pathological thing called the Catastrophic Reaction. What we see is entirely appropriate."

Solms was pointing to the split, the chasm, that marks the different branches of psychiatry. Frustration, tears, and outbursts all seem normal to a psychoanalyst sitting in a room with a man who has lost something as profound as the ability to express himself. But a medical doctor who encounters that same patient might see such behavior in different terms, Solms was saying, might see it in terms of a neurological symptom, "possible explosive anger," for instance, some inappropriate display of emotion that is clearly not "normal." The very contrast between what Silvers sees as frustration and grief, and what a neurology textbook sees as a "catastrophic reaction," demonstrates what psychoanalysis can do for a person like Harry, who might very well not have anywhere else to turn for anything like the same kind of attention and understanding.

"Kindness is probably the basic quality of all therapy," Silvers once remarked to me.

"I feel like kindness is never really discussed so explicitly," I said.

"I feel it should be," he said. "Kindness is major."

In one session, Harry began to cry as he described to Silvers the seemingly never-ending medical treatments he was in the midst of receiving. He pointed to the ceiling, using his characteristic gesture to mean *I might as well die*. He cried a little more, then he stopped, fighting for composure. After a while, he looked pointedly at Silvers. *So?* he seemed to be saying. Silvers looked at him. "I think you will improve." Harry smiled and shook his head.

"Tears, then feeling better. He was in tears and then he was leaving with a handshake. *Thank you thank you*. It's not a cure, but he can go from a mood to another mood," Silvers told me. "So it was a big session."

"Back in the fall, he came in looking dazzling. He really looked good. I said, 'I have to tell you something, Harry. When you come here, you present yourself with a very nice, positive look. It's a pleasure.' *Thank you. Thank you.* Slowly. He took it in. It was no casual thing. Something about that got to him and he felt appreciated."

In his classic collection of case studies, *The Man Who Mistook*

His Wife for a Hat, Oliver Sacks describes an aphasic patient with profound amnesia. Over months of trying to improve his patient's condition, Sacks writes, he came to feel that he had no recourse, no means of helping this man. Nothing he could do would improve his patient's deficits. Finally, at a loss, he wrote to his great counselor, the Russian neurologist Alexander Luria, at that point quite old, to seek his advice. "There are no prescriptions in a case like this," Luria replied. "Do whatever your ingenuity and your heart suggest. There is little or no hope of any recovery in his memory. But a man does not consist of memory alone. He has feeling, will, sensibilities, moral being—matters of which neuropsychology cannot speak." There would be no miraculous breakthrough here, as Sacks had hoped might be possible. Yet ultimately, he concludes, "There remains the undiminished possibility of reintegration by art, by communion, by touching the human spirit."

But the next time Harry appeared in Silvers's office, he was despondent. Silvers had never seen him that way before, slumped over on the sofa, unusually quiet, unable to conjure the motivation to express much of anything at all. That session was the last time Silvers had seen Harry. Throughout our first meetings, Silvers mentioned several times that Harry had yet to be in touch since leaving New York for the winter. It was getting late, Silvers felt. In years past, Harry would have called by now, to say he was coming back soon, could they schedule a time to meet. Silvers debated if and when he should call Harry, whether that would be crossing a line. After all, his patient wasn't obliged to continue the therapy. As Silvers considered the situation, he had a new thought about what had happened at their last session together. Harry's head-down posture might have had something to do with the realization that, tremendously weakened after yet another medical procedure, he was now bound for a full-time life with his parents, giving up the last vestige of normalcy, autonomy, his New York apartment. After ten years of struggling, here was defeat.

"I hope he's alive," Silvers said suddenly, his expression serious.

Behind him, I could see through the door into the neat kitchen, where a fleet of pill bottles lined the countertop, full of the medications Silvers had to take every day.

I didn't yet understand that Silvers's sense of anxiety about Harry's return had plagued him every year when Harry left for his winter hiatus. In fact, I would learn, it often plagued Silvers even from one session to the next. Silvers couldn't quite shake the sense that continuity in the treatment was deeply conditional. "Right from the beginning, my countertransference was that I wouldn't be able to hold him, because somehow, there's not *enough*."

When Silvers attended the monthly group meetings on East Eighty-Second Street, he almost inevitably mentioned to his peers that, despite the connection, the depth of feeling between himself and his patient, he couldn't stop worrying that Harry might not return. "He loves you, you're locked in, he's going to come back," was the group's constant refrain, borne out over years, as Harry kept coming back.

The next time I see Silvers, he is ebullient, appearing brightly at the door and ushering me to the back of the house where we assume our usual positions. Instantly, he makes his announcement. "I'm sitting here like the cat who ate the canary. Why?" he says. Silvers mimes picking up the phone. "*Hello!* The same hello. I said, 'I know who this is!' We talked for a little, in our way. *Thank you thank you thank you*. Meaning, for remembering. You could feel it. It was palpable."

Harry had been calling from Arizona. During the winter, it turned out, a health complication had worsened, and it was now necessary for him to live with his parents year-round. He had indeed given up the New York apartment. Yet the very fact of Harry's interest in continuing the conversation was enough to shore Silvers up, despite the new geographic arrangement and its attendant implication that, in essence, the therapy was over. Silvers didn't see it that way: he was focused on the quality of their connection.

Silvers tried to imagine what they would do now. Maybe weekly phone sessions; maybe they could Skype. Maybe Silvers would go visit him in Arizona. He played with the idea. "I could rent an office space for an hour. We could sit outside." It seemed obvious to me that this would never happen. Beyond the pragmatic concerns, what would even be the point? It would be a breach of the analytic setting, ten times that of going to the ball game, the example Silvers always came back to. More likely: Silvers wouldn't see Harry again. Yet he was buoyant, happy to have Harry back in the fold of communication at all.

"The timing is sporadic, but the tension and the depth are not sporadic," Silvers told me. "The feeling for each other. My concern about him and his concern about me. He says to me, *How are you?* And that's not, how're you. That's, I hope you're still all right because I need you. Or, how are you, I like you. Or how are you, I may depend on you. *How ARE you*. I'm doing very well. *Good good good*."

"I'm still learning," Silvers said, on a different day, on a different note. "The phrase 'how are you.' I'm learning what 'how are you' means. It means you give a damn."

.   .   .

As the summer weeks tick by, Silvers and I continue methodically through the thick pile of Harry's case history. From the beginning, I have felt with Silvers an effortless rapport, an atmosphere that allows conversation to flow and extend in any direction. I understand that the mood in the room, with its quality of humor and warmth, stems from Silvers's own nature, and that to be his patient, I believe, would be to continuously experience this mood, or a version of it, a soft light diffusing the sharp edges of things, lending the voice in one's head an infinitely gentler tone.

"I don't think this particular case warrants interpretation so much as it warrants communication. Now, can we get it to that point where there's so much communication that he says—mumbles— utters—*my sister, no.* The one who died? I don't understand. *No no no.* What did you mean by, 'my sister, no'? But we're not at that point yet."

"It's not analytic in the sense of dealing with unconscious meaning, but it is all from the point of view of an analyst," I say, because I believe I can sense some tremor of anxiety from Silvers on the question of whether or not he is doing "real" psychoanalysis, and I want—appropriately or not—to reassure him somehow.

"We're peeling off the communication problems, a little bit at a time," Silvers replies, nodding. "One day, if you peel enough of the layers, he may say: *my sister, no.* We may get interpretations that are fascinating."

Silvers let Harry dictate their direction more than he might with another patient. He didn't question when Harry stiffened against some line of inquiry. He was careful not to put Harry in the position of having no way to answer what was put to him. Silvers's questions had to be hemmed in like Harry's responses had to be hemmed in. For instance, when Silvers asked about tears from the session before—about frustration—Harry waved Silvers off, as if to say, *We've dealt with that already, forget it.* Silvers didn't pursue it, as he might have with another patient: *Why do you feel that way about it?* Because where would that leave Harry? It would leave him floundering, out of his element, both linguistically and emotionally, and there were too few tools, Silvers felt, to bridge both those gaps at once.

JULY 20, 2009

So we meet again! Last session was almost two months ago. He had a tough July. He was at a movie and had an episode of some kind involving what he could best express as losing his ability to speak—a sort of incoherence—he imitated it with his moving side to side and using his tongue too. Apparently the EMT vehicle came and brought him to the hospital. He was there a few days and his parents came in from the West Coast. For the first time in a long time he pointed up/down about his mood and his parents dying and then he will too, etc. I remarked about this directly. I think the hospital episode has had an effect on his mood, after all it could be very like the stroke of ten years ago, at least emotionally. And his fears of worse things to come are probably somewhere in his consciousness— I believe we alluded to this gently—because I felt it was necessary to face it and express it while we were in session. Then we had to leave and we left at the same time. We'll meet again in September. He seemed fine with the separation—he sort of laughs at me when I assure him, but I'm not so sure this time. We'll see.

.   .   .

I wonder to what extent getting better, for any patient, actually depends on gaining insight. We all have moments of realizing some new truth about ourselves, a discovery that feels, in its revelatory power, as if it should transform the way we go about our lives. And then: it doesn't. Instead, we go right back to normal, armed with our new bit of knowledge. Isn't it possible, then, that insight as such is not the essence of the therapeutic process, that it is not, ultimately, the point? After all, the one constant throughout more than a century of psychiatric practice in all its various forms and ideologies has been the simple fact of two people in a room. Maybe the relationship itself is the point.

19

THROUGHOUT THE SUMMER WEEKS, an imminent happening was on Silvers's mind, and mine too. Mark Solms was hosting his annual conference, three days of the psychoanalysts, psychologists, psychiatrists, neuroscientists, neuropsychologists, neuropsychoanalysts, and other assorted enthusiasts I had come to know in his company, all due to gather this year in Paris. Solms had invited Silvers to present the case of Harry. As the date approached, Silvers was more and more intent on making it there. When I showed up one morning he told me, jubilantly, of what he had just informed his oncologist: "It is only fair that you should know I have plans to go to France."

Silvers was determined to seize the opportunity to show his extended circle of colleagues the possibilities for forging communication and deep connection using the psychoanalytic technique, even with patients who would seem to be so far out of its reach. Yet Ella was frightened for him, after three years of cancer treatment; of the flight, the stress and effort of speaking at a conference, of being in a foreign country. It seemed to me that despite these concerns, Silvers had made up his mind to go and therefore that I would also be going.

On July 3, in a heat wave, I drove to Douglaston to find Silvers in particularly high spirits. The whole country seemed to be on vacation; there was definite indolence in the air. Rather than heading to the back of the house, as usual, Silvers steered me to a little room in the front, a nook, really, and gestured for me to sit down next to him at his upright piano. Messy piles of sheet music covered the top. He was in the midst of teaching himself an old ballad called "How Do You Keep the Music Playing?" I felt slightly awkward, sitting so close together and not knowing quite how to respond to a display so outside of our customary format. But quickly, the pleasure of the music, of the notes ringing out, dissolved my self-consciousness. I requested a few more, and he obliged.

"My hope and wish is to get to Paris. Here's my fantasy: I bring him with me," Silvers said to me when we had moved into the snug little den, our weekly headquarters. Silvers's vision was of the two of them up on stage at Mark Solms's conference, demonstrating for the audience how it was they communicated. Silvers played out the scenario:

"Harry, how you doing today?"

Aaah, nothing, nothing.

"Did you see Sam today?"

Good people, good people, good people.

"How do you like sitting up here?"

Why why why?

"He'd probably be as casual as can be," Silvers told me. "That's *my* fantasy. But I thought you should jot it down because it's a countertransferential thing, that I'd love to show this to people. See this guy who can't speak? Are we having a problem? Apparently not. That's my contribution."

. . .

The next week, back again in the heat wave, I found Silvers abuzz. "Come upstairs for the authentic experience," he said, and we bounded up to the bedroom, hovered next to the unmade bed. "You will not believe this. I've been high ever since." He hit Play on the answering machine.

"Hello, okay thank you and ha-ha-ha. Bye."

The voice was melodic, singsong, and slightly high-pitched; the words issued forth in one continuous stream, with none of the standard pauses and stops, as though they relied on a certain kind of velocity to come at all.

"I'm guessing maybe 'have a happy holiday,'" Silvers said to me, trying to decode the indistinct words. We listened a few more times. There was a sweetness to the voice I hadn't expected. It was a rare exposure to the man himself, tantalizingly real, compared to the elaborate image of Harry I had concocted in my own mind. It was not the first time I had longed to meet him.

For as much time as we had spent discussing Harry, he remained a kind of shadow figure in my mind, except for occasional flashes where suddenly, I believed, I could see this man. I could see him from behind as he painfully, determinedly leaned on the railing to descend the steps into the Seventy-Second Street subway stop, returning home after his hour with Silvers. I could see him gingerly lifting weights at his gym, a former athlete who would now devise any method necessary to get around his injury. But the most enduring picture of all: Harry intently holding the telephone up to his ear, gripping it with his one good hand, on a rare phone call with his teenaged niece—whose mother, Harry's sister, had died a decade before—craving a real connection with the girl, open to it every time, even though he was continually disappointed and hurt by her awkwardness and discomfort with him. These images were nothing more than my own inventions, but they were, in a sense, all I had to go by. I was, at moments, frustrated by the limits of what I could know, worried that I wouldn't ever truly understand what took place between these two men.

20

THERE IS ONE PERSON who has not yet been mentioned, though he has been with us all along. He is Jean-Martin Charcot, the aristocratic French doctor at the heart of Paris's intellectual scene in the last decades of the nineteenth century. He was a dazzling figure. Even through the cobwebs of biography, Charcot retains his sheen. He was impeccable, cultivated, urbane; he spoke and read widely in four different languages. He was the first to identify more than fifteen major neurological illnesses, including ALS (Lou Gehrig's disease), multiple sclerosis, and Tourette's syndrome (though it was named for his student, Gilles de la Tourette). Charcot threw lustrous parties at his house on the Boulevard Saint-Germaine, to which Freud would eventually be invited (and for which he steeled himself with large amounts of cocaine). Charcot had served as the consulting physician for several of the most prominent royal families of Europe. In the 1880s, Charcot, for his professional Act Three, came back to Paris to fulfill a mission at the very hospital where he had first trained: the Salpêtrière, which housed roughly seven thousand indigent women in its sprawling campus in the 13th arrondissement. Here, the patients were awash in all kinds of baffling symptoms, apparently neurological in nature.

By the time Charcot returned to Paris to reckon with it, hysteria had fallen out of medical vogue, because no one had managed to explain it, and the ongoing failure was humiliating for the medical establishment. But Charcot was fascinated by the mysterious syndrome. He put on a public lecture every Tuesday at the Salpêtrière, bringing patients from the hospital wards out onto the stage in front of a large auditorium and guiding them like a magician through a full display of the exotic symptoms that plagued them. It was medicine as theater. All kinds of notable thinkers came to Charcot's *"leçons du mardi"*: the occasion was an intellectual exercise, a literary salon of sorts, with sick people as the stimulation on hand to behold. Scientists and writers came, William James and Guy de Maupassant, and in 1885, Freud did too, in Paris on a six-month fellowship to study under Charcot.

Freud was taken with his new mentor. In a letter to his fiancée, he described Charcot in fetishistic detail:

> At ten o'clock, M. Charcot arrived, a tall man of fifty-eight, wearing a top hat, with dark, strangely soft eyes (or rather, one is; the other is expressionless and has an inward cast), long wisps of hair stuck behind his ears, clean shaven, very expressive features with full protruding lips—in short, like a worldly priest from whom one expects a ready wit and an appreciation of good living . . . I was very much impressed by his brilliant diagnosis and the lively interest he took in everything, so unlike what we are accustomed to from our great men with their veneer of distinguished superficiality.

Solms was riffing on the subject of Charcot and nineteenth-century neurology. We were on the telephone. It was the spring of 2012 and I was calling him from my desk at the news website where I was employed as a science reporter. At the beginning of assignments, I often called Solms, not only for information, but to be instantly transported to the plane of careful thinking he represented to me. No cheap fixes or glib conclusions. Rather: science as process. The best answer we have until we have a better one.

I thought about Charcot a lot when I was with Solms. Both men had been trained in the scientific tradition, yet had knowingly chosen unfashionable, "unscientific" pursuits—Charcot with his hysterics, Solms with his Freud—territories that had already been discarded by the medical establishment, seen as outdated and more than a little unserious. Though Charcot had not found the cure for hysteria, he had set a thousand conversations in motion, revitalizing an ongoing debate about the power of ideas, of the ability of the mind to affect the body. It was Charcot who inspired Freud's creation ten years later of psychoanalysis itself, turning him in the direction of such nonphysical afflictions as hysteria. Of course, when Charcot first took the stage for his *leçons du mardi,* the ramifications were unknowable. He was charismatic and performative, like Solms himself, traits that tend to be looked upon with great suspicion in science. Yet he captured the imagination of the people who heard him and infused their thinking with a new set of possibilities.

"Today we're seeing this amazing promise in the neurosciences," Solms was saying to me on his end of the phone line, somewhere in the southern hemisphere. I pictured him in his silver Volvo, driving along the national highway from city to vineyard, which was what he was often doing when we spoke. "It's where all the brightest minds in science are going, and it's due to the new technologies that have come on the scene in the last few years, like fMRI. But what everyone seems to have forgotten is that we've been exactly here, before: at the end of the nineteenth century, following the invention of the microscope and various staining techniques, neurology exploded with activity. All the brightest minds of those decades, too, flocked to neurology. It really seemed the time was at hand for the mysteries of the brain to be solved. And for three decades, the field stayed like that, right on the cusp, so full of promise— there was a special *glow* over the whole field of neurology. Yet by the end of World War I, not much had come of it, really. Nothing that stuck. And the whole thing more or less fizzled out."

That fall, I was back on the Upper East Side, at the New York Psychoanalytic Institute. Mark Solms was up on stage, declaring that it was necessary to rethink the id. The id, he believed, to the contrary of what Freud believed, is conscious. It is not unconscious. In fact, consciousness *originates* from the id. Solms's idea about the id had come from neuroscience. The clinical implications, Solms admitted, were vast, and he didn't yet have a grip on them.

Solms was up there proposing a major revision to one of the core concepts of Freudian theory. Yet I couldn't help but think that if Freud were here, sitting in one of these polished wooden chairs, he would be enthralled by what he was hearing. Because here we were, more than a century after he scratched out his first formulations about the ego and the id, and his ideas were being batted around with the energy of a high-stakes debate; they were being held up and considered in the light of a whole new scientific field, just as Freud predicted they would be. He always said that what he was putting forward was a working draft, one that he expected and hoped would be revised again and again, down through the generations.

I glanced at the miniature statuette of Freud at the front of the room, just to the right of the stage. This one was cast iron, ten inches tall. Freud was standing in a defiant pose: one foot in front of the other, hands on hips. Somehow, as psychoanalysis evolved, Freud's ideas, indeed, his very persona, became fixed in stone, cast in iron, frozen in place. All the breathing room escaped. Solms and others are engaged in resuscitation and transformation.

None of this is to suggest that the very idea of neuropsychoanalysis doesn't raise its own problems. One person who has given particularly interesting thought to the possible complications of mixing the two disciplines together is Jonathan Lear, the writer, psychoanalyst, and philosopher. For Lear, neuropsychoanalysis is an honorable and worthwhile endeavor in theory, but he cautions about its potential applications. In his book *Therapeutic Action,* he writes: "One has to recognize that however legitimate the interest in neuroscience, there is also a defensive use to which that interest can be put. The defense is to use neuroscience as yet another idealized image of a science that psychoanalysis can latch onto in order to claim legitimacy for itself."

Lear is not the only person to raise the concern that neuroscientific findings might be snapped up by analysts nervous for the future of their profession, waving data from brain research in an effort to fend off public skepticism about the efficacy of the psychoanalytic technique—and, in so doing, cheapening their own artistry.

I had been reading Lear's work for years. His books—on Freud, on psychoanalytic technique, on love, on philosophy, on irony— are conspicuous for their aliveness, their great vibrancy, in a landscape of academic writing that so often feels like just the opposite. I reached Lear by telephone at his office at the University of Chicago. I wanted him to elaborate on his concern about psychoanalysts using neuroscientific findings "defensively." I discovered he had rather a more far-reaching concern as well, when it came to neuroscience, psychoanalysis, and everything in between. Which is to say, the animating assumption throughout much of contemporary neuroscientific research: "Well, that the brain *is* the mind," Lear said.

Oh, right. That.

"Obviously the brain is the organ that supports the mind," Lear hastened to say, "but you know, there's a lot of good philosophical work that shows pretty clearly that simply identifying the brain and the mind just doesn't work."

Lear asked me if I had read a paper called "Individualism and the Mental," by Tyler Burge. Published in 1971, it is a philosophical classic, which illustrates, Lear said, that two people can be in exactly the same brain state, yet still be in two different mental states. That knowing what's happening in a brain, in other words, does not mean knowing what's happening in a mind.

I admitted that I somehow hadn't come across Burge's work.

"You should take that seriously," Lear said. "How could this classic debate be ignored?"

Lear's passion is for uniting psychoanalysis and philosophy. He is surprised, he tells me, that there are not more people doing this. To him, it's perfectly obvious that the two fields belong together, that they ask complementary questions, which is to say: How should we live? How should we be?

"Many neuroscientists would look askance at your statement that the mind is not the brain," I remarked.

"I know, I know," he said.

Tyler Burge's point—and Jonathan Lear's too—is that you can't deal with the brain and expect to therefore not have to deal with the mind. That the two things are not interchangeable. Yet, isn't this exactly the assumption of the studies we encounter, the new, headline-grabbing research we hear described every single day? We might have read, for instance, that the same pathways in the brain that are activated by "love" are also activated by our iPhones (as one study published in 2011 claimed); or that when moments of creative genius come about, alpha waves are emanating from the right hemisphere. What are the guiding assumptions of these studies if not that somehow, by seeing the brain activity correlated with a particular mental function, we are able to understand the mental function itself?

"Something very important was discovered by Freud and worked out in the generations after Freud," Lear continued. "He hit upon some extraordinary therapeutic practices that are very, very special and they need protecting and nurturing. The contemporary culture is not a climate in which they can flourish."

Before we hung up, I asked Lear one final question, directed at his own psychoanalytic practice. "How do you think you'll know when it's time to pay attention to what's coming out of neuroscience?"

"I'm not entirely sure," he answered. "I think the right attitude, and it's the one I try to have, is openness to a future we don't know yet."

21

PARIS IN THE DEAD OF SUMMER: shops closed, humidity thick, neighborhoods quiet, yet laced through with pockets of eternal busyness, Sorbonne students clustered in outdoor cafés talking with energy, smoking with impunity; tourists thronging the banks of the Seine. Jet-lagged, I'm running late to the first day of the conference, which is being held at the Salpêtrière hospital, a sprawling campus of old, short buildings. With my tourist map, I navigate the hospital grounds, a miniature world unto itself, a fortified colony laid down in the midst of the 13th arrondissement.

When I finally locate the building listed on the conference program, I open the doors to an old-fashioned auditorium, dark and cavernous, with rows of uncomfortably narrow hardwood seats and an atmosphere of seriousness, what feels in fact like centuries' worth of seriousness. It isn't until I wander up to the second story later in the day that I discover an enormous mural on the wall, depicting a waifish, otherworldy woman in a floating white dress being held aloft by a small crowd, a crowd that is led by a strong man with a long stick. He is Jean-Martin Charcot, I suddenly guess, which is my first clue that this is the very auditorium where he held his *leçons du mardi.*

. . .

Silvers is in pain. But he is as tenacious, as clear-eyed, as ever. He has come to Paris, taken the long flight with a heartfelt purpose, something like a mission: to convey to all the therapists and scientists of various stripes in the room that this kind of work is possible; that with the most unlikely candidate, a therapeutic connection can still be forged, even outside of language itself. Silvers doesn't regard what he is doing with Harry as remarkable, he has told me many times. Quite the opposite: he sees it as ordinary. Silvers wants everyone in the room to see it that way too, so that they might consider doing something like it, if the chance comes along.

"This is the story of two men," Silvers says from the stage the next day. It is the opening he's had in mind for months. It is the sentiment he most wanted to convey—the humanness, the ordinariness, the deep equality of the endeavor. He had been nervous in the morning, but by the time he takes the microphone, he is utterly in command. He is dressed up, for him, in a yellow button-down shirt, nice black pants, perfectly ironed. He has no notes, but speaks in a spontaneous style, having decided beforehand on the four or five moments from the treatment that he wants to mention. On the projector behind him, he displays one page of Harry's writing. *Six and three quarters,* it says. And: *c-a-s-i-c-s.* It's the note from their first session, when Harry had conveyed how long ago his stroke was, and what movie he had seen that week. (*"Casino Royale,"* Silvers repeats to the Paris crowd.) He describes Harry's personality, being lightly chastised by Harry when he arrived a few minutes late for one of their sessions. He shows one other slide only: the blue-crayon drawing of a man in a rocket ship—the drawing he had done to illustrate his dream, his sense of guilt. "This was a major, countertransferential piece of the whole thing," Silvers explains.

The connection he has managed to forge with Harry is obvious and palpable. It is as clear as anything. Who's to know what ideas Silvers's experience might spark in someone else's mind, someone sitting in this room, I'm thinking. Who can say what new sense of possibility might be opened up. Silvers is joined onstage by two other members of the neuropsychoanalytic group; he is not joined by Susan Ranawat, the psychoanalyst whose patient, Theo, had been so handicapped in a car crash. That treatment had ended sooner than anyone had expected, when Theo's mother moved with him to the West Coast.

I sit next to Ella and take a lot of photographs and feel proud of this man who has given so much of his time to Harry, to me, to his many patients and friends and family, given so much of himself to us all.

Back in New York after Labor Day, Silvers and I return to our reporting process. We continue our weekly meetings, continue to page through the thick file of case notes. At moments, I have the sense that Silvers is stretching out our time, purposefully slowing down our journey to the end of that file. "David as Scheherazade," I jot down in my notebook. We have both become attached to this process. It is about something large and affirming. It is not about cancer. Every week, the pile of what remains becomes ever so slightly smaller. We are moving in millimeters. I don't mind. I relish our hours together, the ease of our connection.

I arrive one day, late in the fall, the crisp air speaking of Thanksgiving, of Christmas. Silvers has purchased thirteen chocolate turkeys and lined them up on the dining room sideboard. He has plans to distribute them with great ceremony to his grandkids when they come for the holiday. We sit down in the den. Somehow, we return again to a subject that's been coming up a lot lately: marriage.

"You wake up in the morning and you look who you're with," Silvers is saying to me with a sudden intensity. He leans forward and looks at me meaningfully. "I'm not talking about beauty. I mean, who are you *with*." Then he leans back again into the sofa cushions and lets silence sit there for a moment or two. He and Ella met when he was twenty, she seventeen. They have been married for fifty-three years.

Silvers and I continue to the end of his thick file, but, as it happens, the last time we meet to talk about the case, it is not the final therapy session we are there to consider, but rather the first: Silvers and I go to the NPAP on Thirteenth Street where there is a file cabinet full of cassette tapes, recordings from meetings of the Edith Laufer group starting in 2006, well before I began to attend. I had wanted to hear Silvers discussing the case back when it was new and he didn't know what he was doing or what he was going to do, didn't know whether it would all come together. I am expecting somehow to find that his attitude will be markedly different, displaying self-doubt or uncertainty; instead I am startled, when we finally get the ancient tape player working, that Silvers has had from the moment this case began an instinctual confidence and determination about the work he is doing. On the tape, he describes to the group the first phone calls, the first sessions, the drama of collecting the small payment. His voice is vibrant and commanding. He couldn't have known how this unusual undertaking would turn out, but he proceeded anyway, with a spirit of openness to whatever might come.

Afterwards, we walk together up Thirteen Street to Sixth Avenue. It has been a brutal winter, and now a tardy spring, and Silvers is bundled up in hat and overcoat, although it is April. It has been more than a year since we began our long conversation. We reach the corner where I turn left and he turns right and we say good-bye. As Silvers disappears up the busy avenue, I have the sudden urge to run after him and escort him through the beastly throngs. Instead, I just stand there and watch him go.

A few weeks later, Ella calls me early one Saturday morning. She knows that I will be attending a small panel discussion that day at which Silvers is scheduled to talk about the case of Harry along with a few of his colleagues presenting their own work. Ella can't make it. Anxiously, she asks me to keep an eye on Silvers. "Of course," I tell her. "How is he doing?"

"I don't know how to answer that," she says. "The cancer is all over his back." She pauses. "But then we've known from the beginning this was just palliative care."

I am stunned, wordless. Silvers hasn't told me, nor in any way suggested, that there is no possibility of vanquishing this disease. On the contrary, I had the distinct impression that his doctors were guiding him towards cure; that this was the aim and intention of the complicated regimen they've had him on for the last three years. Silvers has never hinted to me that he knows he will die from this cancer. Or maybe it's that I failed, utterly, to pick up on those hints, to see, or allow for that possibility.

There is one more question Silvers and I have to answer. We have spent a year talking about the case of Harry. Yet I have never met the man. It has long been my assumption that the story cannot be truly complete without such an encounter. Journalistic logic would put me on a plane to Phoenix, Arizona, to spend an hour or two with Harry, see his apartment, meet his parents, flip through his photo albums, and feel what it is to try and communicate.

Yet when I broach the possibility of such a meeting with Silvers, he is uncomfortable. He has an instinct that it isn't right; but it's only weeks later, on a phone call, that we discuss the issue further. It is the day after the Fourth of July, and I am standing in Central Park when I reach him. All around me, New Yorkers and tourists frolic and laze in the late afternoon sun. "I feel it would be a crossing of wires," Silvers is saying, musing aloud. "And it would leave him confused, like with a certain blankness. He'd probably say to me, *why why why?*"

As Silvers is speaking, it suddenly occurs to me that I don't believe meeting Harry will lead me to a deeper place, will gain me access to a larger truth. For months, I've been immersed with Silvers, trying to understand the process he went through to forge a language with a man who had lost his own. In the end, even in my own story, I don't get to know everything.

ACKNOWLEDGMENTS

Thank you to the whole team at Pantheon who brought this book into existence, especially the great Dan Frank and Betsy Sallee, who made the process a joy. Thank you, as well, to Robin Desser.

Thank you to my agent and dear friend Andrew Blauner, whose help from inception to completion has been unwavering and indispensible.

So many people have generously taken the time to help me better understand their professions. I'd like to say a special thank-you to Joy Hirsch and the Columbia Institute of Psychiatry, Harold Koplewicz of the Child Mind Institute, and Jamshid Ghajar. Thank you to Paula Stahl for urging me in this direction to begin with.

To my magical aunties Peggy, Lesley, and Annie, and to the memory of Dick Grossman, for reading earlier drafts with utmost tenderness and insight.

A huge thank-you to Tina Brown and my editors at *Newsweek / The Daily Beast.*

Thank you to the gang at Neuwrite for including me in many interesting evenings. They have enriched my thinking at every stage of this process. An extra note of gratitude to Armen Enikolopov, who came to check the neuroscience but wound up engaged in many of the book's most central questions.

I am grateful for the existence of the Writer's Room, my sanctuary on Astor Place. Thank you to Donna Brodie for keeping it going and for boosting morale along the way. And as well to my cousin Patti Kenner, who gave me a place to escape the city the many times I needed to.

Many thanks to Beatrice Hogan, for her diligence and precision in fact-checking. I am also deeply grateful to the neuropsychoanalytic steering committee for their abundant generosity.

Thank you to my wonderful friends, whom I treasure, for the intelligence, attention, support, and sympathy, especially Risa Needleman, Jessica Bennett, George Hodgman, Dave Wallace-Wells, Liese Mayer, Aatish Taseer, Judit Somlai, Ariel Schulman, Rachel Smith, Ryan Langer, Zoe Chace, David Sauvage, Chris Nattrass, and Tobias Nolte. An extra blessing on the head of Michael Garfinkle for his fineness of thought about the psychoanalytic material and beyond.

Thank you to my brother Adam Schwartz, whose perspective has helped me out of every kind of jam. And to the rest of my family— my parents, Ernie, Ellie, Zohra, James, and Kat—for their unflagging confidence in what I was trying to do, even when I wasn't sure.

Above all, I am grateful to Mark Solms for saying yes and opening up a world to me, and to the man identified as David Silvers, who added so much heart to mind and brain. He will not be forgotten.

ABOUT THE AUTHOR

Casey Schwartz was formerly a staff writer at *Newsweek / The Daily Beast,* where she wrote about neuroscience, psychiatry, and psychology, among other subjects. Her writing has also appeared in *The New York Times* and *The New York Sun.* She lives in New York City.